Six Parts Love

Six Parts Love

ONE FAMILY'S BATTLE
WITH LOU GEHRIG'S DISEASE

Roni Rabin

CHARLES SCRIBNER'S SONS · NEW YORK

Library of Congress Cataloging in Publication Data

Rabin, Roni.
  Six parts love.

  Bibliography: p.
  1. Rabin, David.   2. Amyotrophic lateral sclerosis—
Patients—Tennessee—Biography.   3. Physicians—Tennessee—
Biography.   I. Title.
RC406.A24R337   1985   362.1'9683 [B]   85-1812
ISBN 0-684-18281-5

The names and descriptions of some people and places have been changed.

A quotation from "Of Dragons and Garden Peas: A Cancer Patient Talks to
Doctors" by Alice Trillin was reprinted with permission from *The New
England Journal of Medicine*, vol. 304, No. 12, pp. 699–701, 19 March 1984.

"Compounding the Ordeal of ALS," by David Rabin, M.D., with Pauline L.
Rabin, M.D., and Roni Rabin was reprinted with permission from *The New
England Journal of Medicine*, vol. 307, pp. 506–509, 19 August 1982.

A quotation from "A Placebo for the Doctor" by Florence Ruderman was
reprinted from *Commentary*, May 1980, by permission; all rights reserved.

To all of the people who helped us wage this battle

Contents

Preface

No one ever forgets his first encounter with ALS. Its deadly initials are imprinted on the minds of all physicians, as they were forty years ago on the minds of the baseball fans who watched the great "Iron Horse" succumb to the ravages of what later came to be called "Lou Gehrig's Disease."

I was a young medical student when I first saw a patient with amyotrophic lateral sclerosis. I had just walked into our Wednesday morning neurology seminar, which was held in a large, cold amphitheater. Down in the pit of the room, on the bare hospital chair that was brought in for "teaching patients," sat a tiny old man. He was stripped to the waist and his skin hung in loose folds around his chest. Where the muscle and fat had wasted away, his ribs were strikingly prominent. He was hunched over in his chair, his face was drawn, and it was painful to watch him strain to lift his arm onto the armrest. He looked sixty-five or seventy years old, and it required no medical expertise to recognize that he was severely depressed.

A few minutes after I came in, our professor, Dr. Smith, entered the classroom. He was a tall, elderly man who had a clipped, sharp manner of speaking, and he exuded very little warmth to his students and even less to his patients. I gasped when Dr. Smith informed us that this patient was only forty-five years old. He then asked the man what his major complaints were. In a barely audible voice, the patient mumbled, "Weakness." After further perfunctory questioning, Smith asked us what we had noticed. A few observant students in the first row remarked that the patient's muscles were twitching, and the neurologist then proceeded to show us the classical combination of "upper and lower motor neuron lesions" that constitutes ALS.

After reviewing the sinister implications of the disease, and the lack of any suitable therapy, Dr. Smith led the patient away. But long after he had left the room, the aura of sadness that the man carried around with him lingered behind. Even the more callous students could not simply dismiss him as "an interesting case." ALS was devastating and demeaning. It was clear that this person had not been given support systems to help him cope with his illness and maintain any semblance of a normal life. Bereft of all hope, he would live out his remaining time in a hospital bed, waiting for death.

The second patient with ALS I saw under very different circumstances. I was a house officer at Baragwanath, a 2000-bed hospital which serviced the entire black population around Johannesburg, South Africa, including the area we know today as Soweto. I had been attending a neurology clinic run by a quiet, humane neurologist called Harry Reefe. I was sitting in his office when he told me that a patient would be coming in shortly.

"You can stay," he said, "but only if you promise not to upset him. He has ALS. I've explained to him in simple language what is happening, and fortunately, he has a daughter who can care for him. But I don't want you jumping up and down trying to elicit a thousand physical signs—all of which he has. It will upset him, and he's got enough on his mind. I'll examine him and arrange for physical therapy if I think it's necessary. Then after he leaves we can talk as long as you like."

What I remember most vividly is the difference in the mental attitudes of the patients. They both had similar physiques, were about the same age, and their diseases were equally severe. Yet that is where the similarities ended; for Jakobus (and it's interesting that I remember his name, though not that of the first patient) was not bowed down and wizened and old. He carried his disease not only with dignity, but also with an apparent greater physical strength which had its source in the compassion of his doctor, and in the corresponding curtailment of the depression which so crushed the first patient.

Five years ago I experienced the first symptoms of ALS. I felt destroyed: I had been an unusually healthy person up until then. Our family life was harmonious, although we had the normal occasional tiffs, and I was doing well professionally. Everything seemed to have come to an abrupt and premature end. I was overwhelmed by shock and depression, and soon my behavior resembled that of the man in the amphitheater. I was biding my time, waiting to die.

This book tells the story of the battle my family and I have waged against despair, frustration, and anger. I made a choice five years ago; it was a choice between despair and hope, between sinking into a quicksand of depression or holding fast to my positive attitude toward life. I made my choice five years ago, but I have made the choice every day since. Every morning I choose to get up instead of staying in bed, to struggle through no longer simple tasks of dressing and washing in order to go to work. I don't get weekends off for good behavior. But there are other rewards; they are the moments of love and laughter I still share with my family and friends, and the sense of satisfaction I get from my work.

This book is written with three audiences in mind. First and foremost, it is dedicated to fellow sufferers, not only of ALS but of other chronic and terminal illnesses. Learning to live with "Creeping Paralysis" has been a difficult process of trial and error; perhaps by sharing my story I can spare others some of my mistakes. As my disease has progressed, my family and I have striven to maintain a constructive lifestyle. Because the presence of chronic illness precludes living a normal life both for the victim and his or her family, we have developed an alternative mode of living which makes allowances for my disabilities and yet is accommodating to the other members of the family. Every time a problem arises we have to find our own solutions; we wish to share our experiences, our coping mechanisms and our shortcuts. Some of our suggestions are pragmatic in nature: they have to do with electric toothbrushes and disposable razors; others are personal and philosophic: they relate to the losses and dependencies consequent upon chronic illness and their impact on the mental health of the family.

In *Illness as Metaphor* Susan Sontag wrote that "Everyone who is born holds dual citizenship, in the kingdom of the well and in the kingdom of the sick." This book also addresses the kingdom of the well. Though the healthy often feel insulated from the tragedy of illness, sooner or later they will come into contact with a chronically ill friend, neighbor, or colleague. How they react may appear to them to be of little significance, but it is crucial to the afflicted family. In ancient civilizations the rules of behavior in this kind of situation were clearly delineated: crippled babies were to be abandoned on mountain tops, aged parents sent out into the snow to die. Today more sophisticated but equally potent forms of ostracism exist. Western society has yet to learn how to incorporate ill people into the general community, and initial responses of embarrassment and confusion, left unchallenged, result in avoidance and evasion of the ill and his or her family.

My family and I have had to contend not only with the grief and anguish of illness, but with feelings of bitterness and rejection. While the former are inevitable, the latter are man-made; hence, both avoidable and unnecessary. To eliminate this bitterness and rejection, communication and understanding are needed on both sides, and I hope this book will be a step forward in bridging the gap between the two kingdoms. That it is possible has been proven by the constant and unfaltering support that we have received from the group of people, some close friends, some formerly mere acquaintances, that have stood by us throughout my illness.

The third audience I would like to reach is the medical community. Physicians are both my colleagues and doctors: sometimes they are fashioned after Harry Reefe; all too frequently they behave like Dr. Smith. The Harry Reefes have been my lifeline. Others of the medical community have gone so far as to change their work hours in order to avoid meeting me. If such people are unable to face up to saying hello to me, how adequate can they be in dealing with the incurable patients who come to see them on a professional basis? They will learn, perhaps, that even when medication is nonexistent and a cure light-years away, there is invaluable therapy that they can always offer their patients, the ingredients of which are support, encouragement, and hope.

—*David Rabin*
June 1984

Acknowledgments

Writing one's first book can be a terrifying experience, and writing this book in particular was an often painful process. I could never have done it without the help of Barbara Koeppel, who gave continuous support and encouragement. I want to thank Ellen Satlow Kapustka and Eleanor Wilner whose perceptive criticism was invaluable, and Diane Vreuls and Stuart Friebert, who taught me everything that can be taught about writing. Eve, Brett, Jim Taylor, Leora Alon, and Ellen gave moral support. My mother Pauline, sisters Dana and Leora and brother Michael, who put up with what I euphemistically called my writer's blocks, are to be commended for their patience and love. For laughs, I depended on Carol, Terri, Cathy, and the Wombat. Most of all I want to thank my father David, who not only inspired me to write this book and shared his story, but also nursed me through difficult periods, poring over the manuscript until together we made a breakthrough or solved a problem.

But there are many other people to whom I am indebted. They are the friends, acquaintances, colleagues, and relatives who have stood by my family during this difficult time. Most of them do not appear in this story because of time and space constraints. To have described all of their lovely gestures would have been impossible. They are the friends who visited from as far away as Australia, and called regularly from as far away as Israel. They are the relatives who came from overseas to lend their support. They are the people, not only in Baltimore but in Washington, Chicago, Toronto, and across the United States, who called, and when David could no longer speak on the phone, who wrote letters. They are the people here in Nashville who came to read to David in the afternoons, and to visit with the family in the evenings. They are the technicians who made it possible for David to continue his research, the secretaries who handled his correspondence, and the doctors who came any time we needed them. They are also the nurses who cared for David, the drivers who took him to work, and all of the service people who did their jobs with grace and sensitivity.

They were our lifeline.

—Roni Rabin

PART 1

The Beginning

CHAPTER 1

Early One Morning

My father David Rabin was always the first one up in the morning. On June 6, 1979, he got up, dressed, washed, and went into the kitchen to make breakfast. His left leg was feeling a bit stiff. He pulled all the breakfast fixings out of the fridge and piled them on the table: jam, cheese, bread, milk, a couple of yogurts, and some peaches. Oh—and a cup of tea set out to cool for Pauli. She would rush in at the last minute, take a few sips and say: "Hey, let's get the show on the road—I've got an eight o'clock patient." David grinned, spread cottage cheese and blueberry jam on a piece of toast, and rubbed his left calf muscle absent-mindedly as he took a bite.

At forty-five David Rabin was a good-looking man with a sensitive face, pale blue eyes and high cheekbones. He was about five feet eight, and slender. But what struck people first was always his accent: After twenty years in the United States he still had a crisp South African pronunciation that Americans found charming. He was articulate and witty; he loved a theory if you had the facts to back it up; he was a good listener because he was interested. Medicine was his main interest, undoubtedly, but classical music, John Updike, Save The Whales—he'd give anything a chance.

It was just past seven. Dana, Leora, and I had no intentions of getting up yet; summer vacation had just started. But Dad liked the cool morning air before the Tennessee humidity set in. He slipped out the back door, opening it just wide enough to let himself out without letting the dogs in. They clambered around him and followed him down the driveway. At the postbox he stooped to pick up the paper. Then he stopped short. His left leg again.

"Oh, hell," he thought, turning left for his morning walk down the street. "It must have been those extra laps I did yesterday." And he put it out of his mind. Unraveling the paper, he skimmed the headlines—no retrospectives on D-Day or the Six-Day War, just the usual sensationalistic stories, so he rolled it up and tucked it under his arm. In the early dawn the green of the trees shimmered with dew. He loved their new neighborhood in Nashville. It was just two miles from Vanderbilt University and the center of town, but it looked and felt like suburbia. The house itself was beautiful—a Tudor style, with ivy creeping up the wooden cross beams, and huge picture windows that flooded the living room with light in the afternoons . . . light flooding through the stained glass windows Pauline had made, beaming through the natural-dye batiks they'd collected from their travels in the Far East, filtering over the African violets Pauli was such a wiz with. Buying the house was one of the crazy, impulsive things they had done, but they'd taken one look at it and known immediately: it was the house they'd always been looking for.

They'd found it just about a year ago. It was about the same time Pauline had started her new job teaching medicine at Vanderbilt, where David was currently chief of the endocrinology department. She had practiced psychiatry for years; she knew people's ins and outs, understood their ebbs and flows. Now she had a chance to share that knowledge—something David had always urged her to do. She was good—the best, he used to tell her, don't keep it to yourself.

David had the feeling it was going to be a good summer. During the past few years the pieces of their lives seemed to be falling together. In a few weeks, Michael would be graduating from college in Chicago, and his graduation gift was a trip to South Africa, the country his parents had left when he was one year old. David was also going back. He had returned periodically over the years to visit his mother, but this trip was a special occasion:

he had been invited to teach an endocrinology course at his alma mater, the Witwatersrand University in Johannesburg. At the end of the street, David stopped to turn around. Funny. The stiffness was still there. It was an unusual feeling. Not so much like a cramp, but more like . . . being on remote control. A short in the system. He wondered if it were a slipped disk. That could account for the stiffness and weakness. But a dislocated disk causes pain. And David had no pain.

He almost wished he did. Because now a strange thing was happening. What David was seeing didn't match up with what he was feeling. The road was flat, but it felt steep. He *knew* it was flat. He was looking right at it; it had only the slightest of an incline. But it felt like an uphill climb!

Back at the house David didn't say anything to Pauline, and by the time they went out to the car, he had almost forgotten about his leg. As chief of the endocrinology division at Vanderbilt he kept a busy day, and today was no different: rounds at eight, a lab meeting at nine, a lecture at ten, clinic all afternoon. And the two of them were meeting at noon for a quick swim during lunch hour.

The morning went as planned, and at ten of twelve David grabbed his boysenberry yogurt from the lab refrigerator and hurried down the hall. But something was holding him back. The elevator door was just about to close and he yelled out, "Just a minute!" and tried to break into a run. But he couldn't do it. He could walk a little faster, but he felt this thing, whatever it was, holding him back. He knew that if he ran he would lose his balance. It was an intuitive, instinctual feeling: if he ran, he would fall. He would just fall flat on his face.

In the elevator he had to compose himself: he didn't want Pauli to notice that he was flustered. Damn it; he was frightened. First the stiffness and now this. Make that extremely frightened. What was going on here?

"Going swimming, Dr. Rabin?" someone intruded on his thoughts.

"Yes . . . thought I'd squeeze in a few laps." Hey, that wasn't a bad idea. The swimming would knock the stiffness out.

"Is everything okay, Dr. Rabin?"

"Sure, just a little preoccupied." And he said to himself, "Snap out of it. Something is happening to me, and it's happening very quickly. But I'm not going to jump to any conclusions."

Down by the car Pauline was waiting for him. Pauline was a short woman, just over five feet three, with an athletic gait that came from tennis and swimming. Her freckles, which disappeared completely in the wintertime, now spread out all over her nose and cheeks. She gave David a smile, showing off her big, white, perfectly straight teeth. As she squinted up to him in the sunlight, her green eyes looked particularly lively, even mischievous. She brushed a wave of short brown hair out of her eyes and said: "Should we walk to the pool today? It's always such a business to find parking for this clunker," and she motioned to the station wagon.

"Well . . ." David answered, hesitating. "I've got a meeting at one, and I've been running around all day. Let's drive—do you mind?"

"Sure doesn't sound like my old Hairbreadth Harry," Pauline said, laughing at the old nickname. Then she added more seriously, "Is anything wrong, Dov?"

"I've just got a little stiffness in my legs," he said. "It'll pass."

But it didn't. Going down the long flight of stairs from the men's locker room to the pool, David had to walk slowly and watch where he put his feet. His eyes were measuring the depth and width of each step, as though they were communicating to his motor nerves, which should have been doing the work on their own. The steps were wetter and more slippery than usual, and he gripped the bannister. "Something is wrong with my motor system," he said to himself. "Very wrong."

Over the next few days the stiffness, which up until now had affected only his left leg, appeared in his right leg as well. Multiple sclerosis. Had he developed multiple sclerosis? Or was it a side effect of the smallpox vaccine he had received in January, before his last trip to South Africa? He had always hated the idea of taking that shot, since he knew that neurological complications resulting from it were far more common than smallpox itself. Even in Africa you have to delve pretty deeply into the jungles to find any traces of smallpox.

But it was all in the muscles! He had no sensory disabilities.

No numbness. No tingling. No pins and needles. None of the running to the bathroom that most MS patients report to their doctors before they know the diagnosis. Only his outgoing motor information was affected—not his incoming sensory information. And in MS both systems are damaged. But again he didn't feel spared. On the contrary. This must be something more specific, less diffuse but more destructive. The only thing he could think of that answered this description was ALS—Lou Gehrig's Disease. But he quickly found reason to push that out of his mind. He had no real weakness. And besides, ALS came on slowly. A person would drop a glass or something, would think it had just slipped and then it would happen again, and again. This was all happening in the course of a few days!

That weekend was hectic. An important contract proposal had to be typed up and sent out by Monday evening. David was one of many who were competing for a National Institutes of Health (NIH) grant of $300,000 to begin his research on a male contraceptive. He had to get cracking. He couldn't be bothered worrying about his legs. Anyway, just a few months ago, he had had a thorough physical exam and had been pronounced in perfect health. How could he have been well one day and now sick the next? It didn't make sense. Of course, the physician in him knew that it did make sense. But this thing had started so quickly, he told himself, it would probably disappear just as quickly. As soon as he stopped thinking about it.

Excuses, excuses. But what psychiatrists call "functional desensitization" or "denial" can be an effective tool, and this time it worked. David reviewed the contract, made a few changes, and found a typist who wanted to make some extra money over the weekend. On Monday he left instructions for his secretary to have the application sent by express mail, and that evening he flew to California for some clinical meetings. He wouldn't have gone except for one thing: there was a conference on a hormone connected to the contraceptive research scheduled for Tuesday, and he wanted to put in an appearance.

The trip was terrible. His flight was delayed; he couldn't concentrate on the journals he had brought with him; to top it off they served ham for dinner. (An abhorrence of ham was one of the carryovers David never shook off from his Orthodox Jewish upbringing.) He had noticed another symptom while walking down the long corridor to his departure gate: if he walked too quickly, the front of his foot would scrape the floor and he would stub his toe. His feet were landing toe-heel instead of heel-toe. Which meant he had foot-drop. Which meant that the ankle muscles were already weak.

David recalled an incident the night before. One of his daughters had touched him and his hand had jumped, as if recoiling from the touch. Sitting in his seat on the plane, he hit his left arm with his right hand to test it. It jerked up. His reflexes were behaving as if they had been bombarded with caffeine or amphetamines. What was wrong?

When the plane landed in Los Angeles, David rented a car and drove straight to his hotel. He was exhausted but felt rejuvenated after a short nap, so he went out and swam forty, fifty, sixty laps in the pool. He skipped all of the meetings except for the conference on LHRH, the hormone he was researching, where he presented some data. Then, an hour later, he flew out of the smoggy city.

The flight back to Tennessee, though it was on schedule, was far worse than the flight out. It was then that David noticed the last symptom, the one he had dreaded most. His worst suspicions were confirmed, because, while sitting in his seat by the window, suspended 35,000 feet above the ground, he noticed that his muscles were twitching.

Twitching muscles is a common enough occurrence. The medical term for it is "fibrillation." On its own it is nothing to worry about. "Benign fibrillation" is a result of too much exercise, or an indication of anxiety. But for David this was just the last in a whole series of signs and symptoms. It was the combination that worried him. The pieces of the puzzle were slowly fitting together in his mind, and he didn't like the picture they were forming. Twitching is associated with only one illness—a deadly, relentless, and cruel disease. This was not benign fibrillation. For while ninety-seven percent of him was still denying vigorously, the remaining three percent knew, without a trace of a doubt, that he had Amyotrophic Lateral Sclerosis.

CHAPTER **2**

One in a Thousand

Amyotrophic Lateral Sclerosis, or ALS, is perhaps the most dreaded neurological illness there is. As it progresses, it produces irreversible paralysis in the patient's entire body, and it may run its course, causing severe disability and death, in a mere three to five years. It is hard to say what a typical case of the illness is. In twenty percent of cases the disease reaches a plateau and patients remain stable for several years. Stephen Hawking, the brilliant British physicist, has lived with the disease for many years while continuing to make breakthrough discoveries in his field. On the other hand, David had read startling reports about patients dying only months after a diagnosis had been made.

The deadly reputation acquired by ALS has made it a pariah in the medical world. For the rest of us, its horror has granted it a protective status of unbelievability and a mythical, almost surrealistic aura. We set it aside, along with natural disasters and freak accidents, as things that can happen only to other people— people we don't know, people who live in small primitive fishing villages on remote islands. ALS is the illness that Woody Allen chose in *Stardust Memories* to explain why he stopped making funny movies, and why, after his friend Bernstein developed the disease, he couldn't find anything to laugh about anymore. Despite the persistent attempts of scientists to discover the cause of the illness, it remains a mystery; no cure or even treatment is known. All that is known is its stealthy and steadfast course, which has earned it the lay names "Chronic Polio" and "Creeping Paralysis."

ALS was first described in the late nineteenth century by a French physician named Dr. Jean Charcot. Forty years ago, it received much notoriety in the United States when Lou Gehrig, the famous "Iron Horse" of baseball, was stricken. Gehrig, a first baseman for the New York Yankees, had a batting average of .340. He had appeared in 2,130 consecutive games; in the course of his career, he hit 493 home runs and batted in 1,990 runs. He was known as the most durable player in U. S. baseball history. But then he started striking out and even dropping the bat accidentally. Soon, he was forced to retire. Confined to a wheelchair, he worked as a parole officer, and when his hands became too weak to write, he dictated the forms to his wife as she filled them out. Months later, he lost his voice muscles; he could no longer speak, chew his food, or swallow. He died at the age of thirty-eight, and ever since his death the illness has been known as "Lou Gehrig's Disease."

David still held out hope that he didn't have ALS. He was an endocrinologist, not a neurologist, but he had almost specialized in neurology so he knew quite a bit about it. He was awfully young to get ALS. Usually it showed up in older people, people in their sixties or seventies. But Lou Gehrig was thirty-six when he was diagnosed, and although ALS is generally considered a disease of the elderly, it also hits children and teenagers. Some studies show a high incidence in David's particular age group, forty-five to fifty-five. David was also banking on the fact that ALS is supposed to develop gradually. He had read about one man who was eventually diagnosed after first presenting his doctor with what seemed like a mild complaint: he couldn't clip the fingernails of his right hand with his left hand. Whatever David had wasn't wasting time with such niceties!

But David knew the symptoms. He could hear his neurology professor of twenty-five years ago, speaking as if it were yesterday, about "the classical combination of upper and lower motor neuron lesions." It was precisely this classical combination that was causing these strange symptoms. The upper motor neurons, or pyramidal tracts, lead from the brain to the spinal cord. The lower motor neurons, or anterior horn cells, continue from the spinal cord to the muscles all over the body. Nerves are messengers; when they're damaged the communication is cut off between the brain and the limbs. The muscles don't get their commands; they weaken and atrophy. "The patient describes feelings of weakness and stiffness. . . ."

And twitching! Electrical activity is generated in the muscles, but in order for it to be effective, it must be shaped and coordinated by the nerves. When the nerve isn't there to restrain and direct the electricity, it goes wild. It can happen in a few individual fibers, and then it looks like twitching on the surface of the muscle. That is because of damage to the lower motor neuron. When a whole group of muscles shakes up and down and a whole limb is affected, it is a result of damage to the upper motor neuron and is called clonus.

David knew he needed another opinion. A doctor should never make his own diagnosis, especially in a case like this. There was too much at stake. All attempts at objectivity were shot. Besides, he had left neurology years ago. He never knew exactly why he had left, it had just happened; he had found studying hormones and glands more enticing. But now he realized why. It just clicked all of a sudden. The hopelessness. Neurology was such a depressing field. The professors used to say, "There are only twelve curable diseases in neurology. So when you get a patient, first look for those twelve. After that just sit back and take your time. There's nothing you can do anyway." Nerves are the image of delicacy: thin fibers dangling, like pieces of cotton or spider's threads, so vulnerable to bones and surgeons' knives and automobile accidents; and once chopped down, irreparable, broken forever. Hopeless. "Nerves don't regenerate"—the basic axiom of neurology. Surviving nerves, in a process known as collateral sprouting, may be able to take over the territory of damaged nerves, thus enabling a group of muscles to continue functioning. But once the nerve cell body is killed, that's it. It will not regrow. So what did a neurologist—any, the best in the world— have to offer David now? Hope. That was all he could expect. And he was already hoping as fast as he could.

He was hoping he had a disease that mimicked ALS. He had no weakness, remember? Only stiffness. And ALS was so rare, something like one in one hundred thousand. Actually, it hits one to three of every one hundred thousand people in any given year. At any point in time, six to seven out of one hundred thousand people are suffering from the illness. But this had developed so quickly; And ALS came on slowly, insidiously, although some of the books did say that it could manifest itself in sudden jerky "fits and starts"—erratic but distinct. . . .

In the next few months, David would memorize many irrelevant statistical data about the illness—irrelevant because they shed no light on the cause or cure of the illness. For example: more men are affected than women, with a ratio of 1.8 to 1. But no one has any idea why. Fifty percent of patients die within three years, some during the first few months of the illness. In others the disease appears to reach a plateau after two or three years and goes into complete or partial remission. Twenty percent of patients survive for five years or more; ten percent live for ten, fifteen, and sometimes twenty years with the illness. *But there is no regeneration of the already damaged nerves.* And in a few isolated places in the world, in western New Guinea, the Kii peninsula of Japan, and among the Chamorro people in Guam, the incidence of ALS is a hundred times higher than anywhere else in the world. Again, no one knows why. Scientists have compiled reams and reams of data; studied genetic traits, environmental factors, racial origins—and they haven't come up with anything. No clues. Nothing. Hopelessness.

Not to panic. Not to panic. Three magic words David repeated like a mantra. You haven't even seen an expert. Not to panic. Keep your cool. Not to panic. Don't want to ruin Michael's graduation weekend in Chicago—not to panic.

When he got back from California, the first thing David did was go swimming. He was convinced that he could swim this thing out, work it out, exercise it away. He dug the dumbbell weights out of the basement and called the hotel in Chicago to check if they had a pool. They didn't. He canceled the reservations and found a hotel that did. He borrowed a stationary bicycle from some friends and put six miles on it that very night. He already knew he was going to fight. He figured that even healthy muscle will atrophy if it sits still. So he decided on a strict exercise regimen. He was going to build up all the muscle he could.

By now he was dragging his left leg. He looked terrible, the worry showing through on his face. And his left leg, hanging limply, gave the impression that his whole left side was paralyzed. He looked like he had had a stroke. People kept asking him what was wrong, and he kept saying that it was from moving the couch last weekend, and that he must have pulled a muscle in his back.

Mom wasn't really worried at the beginning. Of course, she felt bad, since it had been her idea to change the furniture around. But Dad never got sick. He was like Lou Gehrig that way; he never missed a game. In the twenty-three years that my parents had been married, he had never gotten sick. It was Mom who got the terrible flu every winter, Mom who had the hepatitis that cold winter in London, Mom who had mysterious lumps and aches. And he took care of her. Those were the roles they played; and no one changes the rules in the middle of the game.

A few days later, Dad told us that he had dislocated a disk, and though our opinions varied as to how he should approach the problem, we never stopped to question the basic premise. I was nineteen. I had just finished my sophomore year at Oberlin, and I really believed that all the ills in the world could be cured if people pulled together, worked hard, and helped one another out. Provided they had the right priorities, of course. No, I wasn't naive, I would argue; idealistic. My sister Dana was fourteen—five years younger than I. Dana's reaction was immediate denial—it's just a bad back; we'll take care of it and it will get better. Of the three of us, my sister Leora was the most realistic, even though she was only thirteen. Dad told me later he thought she had known somehow from the first. He caught her cocking her little head to one side, squinting at him, as if she were trying to see through the glare. And she didn't hesitate to voice her opinion.

"Well, why don't you see a doctor, Dad? You think you're so smart you don't have to see a doctor?" she yelled at my father.

"Yeah, why don't you go see someone, Dad?" I backed her up.

"You guys, hey you guys," Dana interrupted. "You don't know anything. My friend Joanne's father had a disk and he's com-

pletely okay now. I mean, he had it for a long time but now he's
okay and he doesn't limp anymore. So just don't get upset and
worried about it 'cause it's not that terrible."

We didn't really need Dana to convince us. The truth was that
none of us were very worried. After a few days, Dad's color was
back to normal, and though he was still dragging his leg, we had
accepted the explanation he gave us. We didn't think about it
very much. Like most people, we had never heard of ALS. We
had no reason to associate this slight limp with the wheelchairs
on Muscular Dystrophy Association pamphlets or posters of fund-
raising carnivals. Bad backs, like wrinkles and arthritis, were one
of the unavoidable hazards of aging. Even later, as the disease
progressed, we didn't make the connection. Some things are so
threatening, you don't even imagine them. You might dream them
in a nightmare, but you don't match them up with the evidence
in broad daylight. I didn't even wonder about it. It wasn't an
option. A back problem and a life-threatening illness are two
different issues altogether; Dad was neatly tucked away in one
category—if anything, the slipped disk gave the illusion of safety.
"There, he's had his share of problems."

That Friday Dad was still on Hairbreadth Harry time, and we
were supposed to pick him up at the hospital at noon and leave
from there for Chicago. At eleven he gave a lecture to the third-
year Vanderbilt medical students. When he finished speaking and
turned to leave the podium, a strange thing happened: he suddenly froze. The freeze didn't last more than a few seconds, but
for those few seconds he couldn't move. Not a finger. He tried to
step forward, but he couldn't. He just stood there and held on to
the lectern. Then it passed.

The four of us were waiting for him in the car. We were all
packed and ready to go. He was a few minutes late, but we
expected that, since the limp slowed him down. He swung himself
into the front seat and said, "Okey dokey, we're on our way!"
and then we were off. We passed around tunafish sandwiches and
potato chips, and then we settled back in our seats. Everything
was going as usual. No hitches. Dad drove the whole nine hours
up to Chicago. Michael came to see us at the hotel that night,
and then Dad went for a swim. The next morning the graduation
ceremony was held on the lawn. It was sunny and dogwoods were

blossoming. In the pictures everyone was smiling. I didn't know that that night while Michael went out with his friends, and Dana, Leora, and I were watching TV in our hotel room, Mom and Dad were at a little cafe having a talk. I only found this out two years later, when Dad and I spent whole mornings reconstructing the events for this book. Apparently, Mom forced the issue—she knew it was serious, she told him. It could be a tumor of the spinal cord on the left side. Or worse. He must see someone right away. They both agreed to keep up the pretense in front of us children. And when they got back to the hotel they went for a midnight swim. Swimming was supposed to be excellent therapy for slipped disks.

CHAPTER 3

The Doctors

Monday morning, after we'd returned from Chicago, David called Dr. Elliot Fitzgerald. He'd like to see him professionally, he said. It's nothing serious, he said, really. But if Fitzgerald were busy during the week maybe he could just see him on a Saturday or Sunday? He'd been having some symptoms . . . he'd like a neurologist to examine him.

Fitzgerald said, fine. He was a man of medium height, with green eyes and dirty-blond hair. He wore straight-legged pants and penny loafers with pennies in them. David had heard he was a competent clinician, even more than competent. They had met several times at parties, and had exchanged small talk at medical gatherings. But it had been several months since they last spoke.

On Sunday David met Fitzgerald in his office. He listed his symptoms: stiffness in his legs, hyperactive reflexes in his arms, fasciculation. Only he didn't use the term "fasciculation"—it was too condemning a word. He said his muscles were "restless." He had been abnormally tired after his trip to California, he said, and he was dragging his left leg.

"Those signs are all very subtle though," Fitzgerald said in a monotone that wasn't too reassuring. "Very subtle. I wouldn't get that worked up about them. You know people's muscles twitch from fatigue sometimes. Have you had any weakness?"

David shook his head, no. He'd conveniently forgotten about the foot-drop.

"Well, let's start off and test your strength. Here, grab my hands. Squeeze them as hard as you can . . . that's pretty good. Okay, now, hold out your arms and cock your wrists up . . . now, with me holding them down try it again, just push up against me . . . okay. Now, bend your elbow and I'll try to restrain it— just push up against my hand. Now, straighten it while I'm pushing the other way. Great . . . now I'm going to hold your forehead up, and try to bend your head forward against my hand. Okay, I'd say you're doing pretty well. There's no sign of weakness that I can detect, you're actually quite strong. Any problems with your facial muscles at all? Try clenching your teeth . . . smiling . . . frowning . . . can you hold it? . . . good. Close your eyes, keep them shut . . . pretty good.

"Let's take a look at your reflexes now." Fitzgerald pulled out a small reflex hammer and gave a little knock on the shoulders, on the elbows, on the forearms, the hands, the thighs, lower legs, chest . . . everywhere. And everywhere he knocked responded with a jerk upwards, a jump, a twitch of the muscles. Abnormally brisk reflexes all over, which both of the doctors saw and which both knew to be signs of upper motor neuron damage. The pyramidal tract, whose task it was to dampen the effect of the hammer's stimulus, was not functioning correctly; the stimulus continued unrestrained, back and forth and back and forth. But Fitzgerald didn't say anything; he just avoided David's eyes.

The other thing doctors look for when testing for upper motor neuron damage is the so-called Babinski response. The Babinski is a funny test: the doctor strokes the soles of the patient's feet with an object, like a car key, and watches the toes. If they curl downward everything's okay; if they curl upward that's an abnormal response. David's toes curled down.

Now Fitzgerald tested David's sensation. "Close your eyes and tell me what this feels like," he said, rubbing a ball of cotton on David's cheeks.

"Cotton wool."

"Right. Can you feel this now?" Fitzgerald continued, pricking David lightly with a pin.

"Ouch—yes!"

"Okay, what am I doing now?"

"Holding my toe up."

"And now?"

"Holding it down."

"Good." Fitzgerald took a tuning fork, knocked it, and held it against the joint in David's left big toe. "Tell me when the vibrating stops."

"Okay . . . now."

"Right. Terrific. You can open your eyes now." Fitzgerald now took David's left foot and bent the ankle up to a ninety-degree angle. Then he let it go. But the muscle did not stop. It just kept going on and on, up and down and up and down, six or seven times.

"Okay, I think that'll be all for now, David. Why don't you get dressed. Listen, I, uh—I don't really think it's all that serious. You don't have any weakness or any sensory dysfunction . . . and you've got a negative on the Babinski."

"What about my reflexes?"

"Well, they're very brisk, very brisk, no doubt, very quick. But they may have been like that for the past few years already, and you just haven't noticed it until now. It could just be a chronic sort of thing." Fitzgerald was being evasive. He couldn't bring himself to look at David; instead he paced up and down the room, and when he got to the window, he stopped and stood there, staring out into the parking lot.

"I can't just ignore this, Elliot," David said. "I have to find out what's going on. You may not think it's serious, but, hell, I'm forty-five years old and I wake up one morning and I can't run. I've been in perfect health, I swim every day, and suddenly there's this thing. . . ."

"I don't really think it's that serious," Fitzgerald said impatiently, in a tone to stop all conversation.

"What do you *mean*?" David asked, incredulous. "Damn it— I can't run. I'm healthy and suddenly I just can't run, and you don't think it's serious?"

Fitzgerald shook his head. He was being very cautious. He was not just going to tell a man, on the basis of twenty minutes of observation, that he had a fatal illness. And besides, he was embarrassed. David was well versed in neurology himself; he was a world figure in endocrinology. Fitzgerald didn't want to pass a verdict on this man. He didn't really want to say anything.

He didn't want to get involved. The thought of dealing with an ill person . . . of dealing with himself dealing with an ill person . . . made him recoil. More than anything, he just wanted to pass the buck.

"I don't know what to tell you," he said.

"Okay, then. I'll tell you what you can tell me. Who's the expert in this area? Who knows the most? That's whom I want to see. The best. Can you find that out for me?"

"That I can tell you right now. Dr. Fields. At the UCM clinic."

The next day David called the UCM. A secretary with a sing-song voice answered the phone. "I'm sorry, but Dr. Fields is all booked up for . . . let me see here . . . the next six months. I can put you down for December 13, and we will call you if there's a cancellation before then . . . should I do that, sir?"

"No." David hesitated for a moment. He just couldn't wait that long. "Do you think I could speak with Dr. Fields for a moment? Is he around?"

"Just one moment please," the singsong answered.

"Dr. Fields here. Can I help you?" A loud voice came over the line.

"Yes, you certainly may, Dr. Fields. How are you . . . my name is Dr. David Rabin and I'm at Vanderbilt University in Nashville. Dr. Elliot Fitzgerald recommended that I see you. I've had some very worrying symptoms, indicating ALS. Your secretary tells me that you're very busy, but I can't wait until December. I need a definite diagnosis. Could you possibly find a slot for me in the next few weeks?"

"Yes, certainly, I understand perfectly," Fields answered. "I'll fit you in next week. David should prepare for five days of tests and examinations.

CHAPTER 4

Test Results Only

The UCM clinic is a large medical center that dominates the small town. Everyone who lives in the town either works at the hospital or at one of the many businesses that service the medical center: restaurants, motels for visiting patients and their families, laundromats. Almost everyone who flies into the tiny airport on the outskirts of the town is going there for medical reasons. They travel for hundreds of miles, and they don't make the journey lightly. Some depend on walking aids to get on and off the plane; they have trouble getting down the aisles. Many of the women wear scarves over their heads where the hair has fallen out from chemotherapy treatments or brain surgery. These people come to consult specialists, to get advice, to hear about the newest research, the latest successful treatment. Most of all, they come to get some hope.

The UCM is run very efficiently and operates almost entirely as an outpatient facility. This saves a lot of money for everyone involved. David had expected to take all of the tests as an inpatient, since most hospitals don't have the ambulatory facilities for outpatient testing, and try to keep their beds full for financial reasons. Not so here. David checked into a hotel across the street from the hospital. It cost forty dollars a night, as opposed to the one hundred sixty he would have paid for a hospital room. He ate lunch in a small restaurant down the street instead of in the hospital cafeteria. And at two o'clock he went in to see Dr. Fields.

Dr. Fields was a tall, well-built man with a broad face. Everything about him suggested his being solidly rooted, stable, and sure of himself. He had an aura of command, an authoritative presence: Fields knew ALS inside out. But he was very distant, and David got the distinct impression the distance was premeditated and deliberate. All of Fields's actions were calculated and intentional. His office was immaculate; his books were arranged alphabetically by author. When David came in, he was sitting behind a large desk. After a brief handshake and a perfunctory "How are you" he got straight to the point.

"I take it from our telephone conversation that you are familiar with the disease. You are almost certain of the diagnosis already. We'll do a clinical exam and then an electromyograph. Is there anything you'd like to ask me before we begin?"

"Yes," David started, leaning over in his seat, "I'll be quite honest with you. I came here for three reasons. I want a definite diagnosis. But I also want to know what to do—I want to hear what research is going on, particularly with plasmapheresis, and I'd like to know something about the etiology of the disease, and what physical therapy might be helpful. And the third reason I came here was . . . I want some hope."

"Okay," Dr. Fields said, "I'll try to help you, as much as I'm able. Why don't we start with you going over the symptoms from the beginning."

Once again, David repeated his story. Fields listened, nodding as he jotted down notes on a large yellow pad; then he asked a few questions.

"Have you had any weakness?"

"No, just stiffness."

"You're sure?"

"As far as I can tell."

"Good. Any pain?"

"No. Some cramping in my muscles, but no pain."

"Think carefully. Any back pain, pain in any part of the leg or foot?"

"No . . . none at all." David realized that Fields, too, was trying to find evidence of a dislocated disk.

"Okay. Let's try a few things. Can you hop across the floor on one foot? Go ahead, try it."

David tried. He could hop on his right foot, but not on his left. "Why don't you get undressed. We'll do a physical exam and see how you walk without shoes and socks," Fields said.

But without the shoes operating as splints for his foot-drop, compensating for the loss of muscle in his ankles, David had great difficulty getting across the room. Then Fields stabilized David's left wrist and said, "Now. Try to flex your hand. All the way. Can you get it any further out? Try to flatten it. Any more? Let's see the other hand."

He repeated the exercise one more time, but David couldn't stretch his fingers out all the way if Fields was holding his wrist down.

"You see—that's where the weakness is," the expert said, with a note of pride in his voice. "You have so many hundreds of muscles that you can easily compensate for the loss of one with another one close by. Trick movements like that conceal the weakness and the wasting of muscles that's taking place."

It was very simple: Fields knew what to look for. In the space of a few seconds he had identified the lower motor neuron damage: weakness and paralysis. He told David to sit at the end of the couch and try to pick his feet up off the floor. He could tell, by feeling the tendons around the ankle, that the muscle was not contracting as much as it normally would, nor were the tendons as taut as they should be.

"One more time: you have no pain?"

"Right."

"Pins and needles?"

"No."

"Any problems controlling your bowel movements or your bladder?"

"No."

"Sexual problems? Any impotence, for example?"

"None."

Fields wasn't one to procrastinate. He'd seen hundreds of patients with degenerative nerve disease, and he rarely made mistakes.

"As far as I can tell from a clinical exam," he said, "it looks like ALS." He used the same tone of voice a handyman would use to tell you that your gutters were full of leaves and had to be cleaned out before the next major rainfall.

David stayed at UCM for a week. He kept hoping they would find something—anything. Anything would be preferable to ALS. Multiple sclerosis at least has periods of remission; it comes and goes, and people live with it for years. Even cancers are treatable— it's a battle, but at least there's a chance. Radiotherapy and chemotherapy are far from pleasant, but at least there's something to hang on to, something to hope for, reasonable odds for a gamble, a fighting chance. But every day another unknown variable was identified and uncovered, and each only served to confirm the hypothesis. There were blood tests, urine tests, a lung function test. David had an appointment with a gastroenterologist to check for rectal cancer. By now rectal cancer would have seemed like a blessing. In between the tests there was a lot of free time, time to go crazy if he wasn't careful, time to wish he had brought Pauline along with him even though it would have aroused our suspicions. He swam twice a day, in a pool at the motel with all of the other desperately ill people. He walked a lot, from one side of the little town to the other, back and forth and up and down the streets of the city. One evening there was an outdoor concert in the park, and he listened from the road as he walked up and down for an hour and a half—anything to keep on using those muscles, to keep on walking. And at night he called Pauline to fill her in on the details of the latest tests. The lung function was the only one Fields had shown him: it was the only one with normal results. But that was crucial because the heart is not affected in ALS, and when people finally die it is usually from respiratory difficulites.

The EMG was the final test, the conclusive test, the one which would provide a definitive diagnosis. In an electromyograph a needle electrode is inserted into the muscle. The needle is connected to a machine that monitors the amount of electrical activity in the muscles. If the patient has ALS, the monitor will register a pattern of abnormally high electrical potential called "denervation." The criterion for ALS is that denervation be found in at least three of the patient's limbs. This rules out the possibility of a local syndrome, such as a tumor, being the cause of the abnormality.

The intern performed the test on three of David's limbs. Then he stopped. "I think we're through," he said, "but I'm just going to check with Dr. Fields to make sure."

The moment he left the room David knew it was all over. The intern must have found denervation in all three limbs. Otherwise he would have gone ahead and done the fourth limb automatically.

David had several conversations with Fields during this time. They discussed the possible causes of the illness, and Fields told David about ALSSOA, the Amyotrophic Lateral Sclerosis Society of America that puts out a monthly newsletter and sponsors research all over the country. David thought it curious that Fields didn't ask him any personal questions—whether he had a family, what he did at Vanderbilt, what his financial state was, whether he would be able to continue working once he became physically disabled. And Fields didn't volunteer information either. David prodded, but Fields maintained his cool reserve.

"What kind of shoes should I wear?" David asked.

"Oh, anything that's comfortable," Fields answered. But that was ridiculous: David had foot-drop. He needed a shoe that would support his ankle, yet not be too heavy. He needed the kind of sole that wouldn't catch on synthetic carpets and fluff, and make him trip.

"What do you think about my going to South Africa this summer?" he asked.

"Listen, if you're up to it, go," came the answer.

"Well, I'm not sure if I'm up to it. I feel all right on the whole, but it is a seventeen-hour flight and it means being away from the family and Pauline. . . ."

"See how you feel in a couple of weeks."

"Okay. One last thing," David said. He was becoming extremely frustrated. "What's your feeling about exercise—can it help? Can it hurt? My theory is that if I don't exercise I'll be compounding the wasting process which is occurring anyway. I want to know what your opinion is. Swimming seems like it could be a good help. What do you think?"

Fields just shrugged. He didn't say anything but the message was clear: Hell, I don't think anything helps. He ended the interview by saying, "Listen, make an appointment with my secretary to come back and see me, say, in three months' time. She'll find you a slot."

"Okay, thank you." But David knew he wouldn't be back. He had nothing to gain from a repeated visit. He could see for himself if the disease was progressing, and Fields promised no more than that. He had come to Fields asking for a definite diagnosis, but also asking for some therapy and some hope. Fields had given him a diagnosis.

CHAPTER 5

Hey Lady You Don't Know Disaster

David hid his grief the same way he hid his weakness, with trick movements. He told us he'd been up in Michigan working on some research with a friend. After dinner, as we watched the news together, he went through the motions of being excited about one story and irate about the next. But he didn't really care; his act was for our benefit only. As far as he was concerned, the world could take its revolutions and arms limitation treaties and presidential elections and just go to hell. He had ALS. He was going to die.

He thought he would die very quickly. A couple of weeks, maybe months. If the disease continued to progress as quickly as it had gotten started, it would be no time before it crept up into his thorax and his chest. It was already there in his arms, where the EMG needles found it. He remembered seeing an article about a woman who died a month after the diagnosis was made. He tried to get his papers in order—he and Pauline went into the hospital to clean out his office, file the journals, return overdue books, complete manuscripts, answer letters. Most people wonder, "Why me?" but he wondered, "Why *this*?" Why not a heart attack, a cancer? Of all the diseases in the textbook, why this one? Creeping up on him. Eating away at him every day.

He pulled himself together enough to go to work. His work had always played a central role in his life. He had never been a nine-to-fiver, rather, he put in ten hours, sometimes eleven and almost twelve, and then after dinner he read the medical journals to catch up with the latest breakthroughs and ideas. His interests weren't confined to one area of medicine: he taught, and students flocked to his classes because of his clear, concise explanations, as well as his jokes (on infertility: Why do the Chinese limit families to one child each? Because otherwise it would be a gang of four). In the lab he was a perfect technician, getting in there with the test tubes and antibodies and using creative leaps of the imagination to figure out the next step in an endocrinology experiment. In the hospital, by the bedside, his patients loved him because his reputation gained their confidence and his gentle manner indicated genuine concern for their fertility problems.

David had relied on his work to get him through tough times in the past. Now, for the first time, his grief and shock were too overwhelming to be absorbed by his work. He kept going in to the hospital. He never missed a day. But he had to feign compassion for his patients. A woman came into the fertility clinic crying because she couldn't conceive another child—she had two already, but they wanted a third: "Please, doctor, isn't there anything you can do? A pill, a shot, anything." Another woman had mild hirsutism on her face. A little down on her lips, her chin. "I can't live like this," she said. "Look what I look like. Disastrous. I'm so miserable, I'll do anything. My whole life, my love life, in jeopardy." David examined the women and spoke quietly to them. He listened and tested and prescribed. But all the time he was thinking, "Hey, lady, you don't know disaster. Hey, lady, you don't know jeopardy."

David didn't go through the five stages of grief described by Elisabeth Kübler-Ross. What he went through was inchoate and formless. Chaotic. There was no orderly process, no neat steps to go through one by one. He was suspended in a vacuum, removed from everything he used to love and care about. He had no enthusiasm, no motivation to do anything; he was listless and lethargic. At night he couldn't sleep, almost as if he was so horrified by death that he couldn't even surrender to its benign cousin. Pauline, on her side of the bed, would strain her ears to listen: is he breathing? If she could hear him snoring softly the

safety of the rhythm would rock her to sleep. Otherwise she lay
awake, tense and alert, listening.

And David lay there thinking. He planned the funeral over and
over again in his head; counting the mourners, writing the eulogy
for the rabbi. He became obsessed with the arrangements. He must
remember to tell Pauli that he wanted to be cremated. And the
music: they must play the Brandenburg concertos and the Beatles.
Yesterday. Seemed to fit him so well. "Yesterday, all my troubles
seemed so far away . . . now it looks as though they're here to
stay." Losing his health was like losing a lover. He had always
appreciated her and treated her well so that she would stay. Never
taken her for granted. On his last birthday he remembered having
the thought, "Gosh, I'm forty-five already," and then, almost in
the same mental breath, "And I'm healthy." He had never been
an envious person, but now he experienced jealousy. He was
jealous of people—not because of their brains or their money,
but their health. Their independence. Their future. He had looked
forward to middle age, with the kids out of the house and more
time to spend with Pauline. To relax, travel. There were good
aspects to aging—security and professional recognition. Compared to what awaited him now: he would have to be dressed,
bathed, fed. He felt like he had woken up inside someone else's
fate, and because he was in there the rest of the family was in there
with him. Just the thought that Dana and Leora wouldn't have
him around to solve their chemistry problems—or Michael and
I, to discuss income tax returns—made him want to cry. And then
he imagined us, all alone. Pauline, coming home to an empty
house. Doing the accounts all alone at the end of the month. A
gray overcast light in the kitchen, where she sits at the table with
a pile of bills. . . .

Then, finally, he would fall asleep. Get a little rest. But he
would wake early, at three-thirty, covered in cold sweat. And he
would hear the crickets and the birds outside in the early dawn
and then he'd remember: it's not a nightmare. It's for real. I'm
not going to wake up to find this all over. Every time I wake up,
it's going to be there, waiting for me. It's me, and it's our little
family. The six of us, pulling through. And then he'd think of all
we'd been through already. Little Lisa dying before she was six

months old, in a small flat in Baltimore in the Sixties when he'd been on the faculty at Johns Hopkins Medical School. The trauma of all the moves—to Israel in the late Sixties, then back. The guilt about leaving Israel. Finally settling in Nashville, where things looked like they were calming down a bit, finally working out, running smoothly . . . now this. Why now? Why this? Why us?

Four o'clock. Pauline heard the bed springs creak as David tossed. "Dovi?" she'd whisper. And she'd talk to him softly, and she'd soothe him. "Dovi, you can't sleep, you're so anxious. And it's natural, it's normal for you to be anxious and depressed with this terrible news. Why don't you get up and go downstairs and make yourself a cup of hot chocolate. Then go ride your bike. Use your muscles and while you're using them you'll feel better because you're building them and fighting the wasting." Pauline honestly believed this; it was the only thing that kept her going.

So the two of them would slip downstairs, tiptoeing past Dana and Leora's bedrooms and into the kitchen where David asked her, for the fifteenth time in twenty-four hours, whether he should make the trip to South Africa or not.

"I think you want me to make the decision for you, Dov, and I can't, I just can't do that. If you go I'll be worried about you. I guess I don't really want you to go, I'm so scared, but it might be your last chance to see your family. . . ."

"What's going to be hardest is that I—Well, I was always the big shot. Not the big shot exactly, but they looked up to me. I was the one who got the scholarships to medical school, I was the one who became the doctor and got out of the retail business, I went to America and became the big professor. They always came to me to find out what their doctors were doing and to get my advice . . . I always had a solution to everything. The candy man. 'Go ask Uncle David, he'll tell you what to do.' Now, all I have is a big, fat, utterly insoluble problem. I just don't know if I can face them."

"What did Fitzgerald say about it? You talked to him, didn't you?"

"Oh, he just shrugs his shoulders. At anything I say. I'm as good as dead already in his book. When I told him the diagnosis was confirmed, he said, 'You know, this is the fourth time I've

seen such a young person with ALS and every time it's so traumatic.' For him. For him it's traumatic! He should see how it
feels on this end! He acted like he expected me to apologize for
having this disease because it put him in the uncomfortable position of having to diagnose it. Christ! I've got it. I've got to live
with it." And die from it, David thought, but didn't say.

He would have preferred a heart attack. Wham, bam, and it's
over. It's a snap. Don't think about it ahead of time, never know
when it's coming. Though of course he'd heard stories of widows
whose husbands had died like that. Suddenly. Out of the blue.
They didn't know where the papers were, what the name of the
lawyer was, how much money was tucked away in bonds and
policies.

"Did you discuss your exercise program with him?" Pauline
asked, hopefully.

"Well, it's always good to keep your muscles in tone," David
said, in a sarcastic tone of voice.

"What do you mean?"

"That's what he said. 'Well, it's always good to keep your
muscles in tone.' How's that for encouragement? He might as
well have said, 'Don't waste your time, you haven't that much to
waste.' I asked him to look up some articles about plasmapheresis
for me. What is it about neurologists? They're so cold and
impersonal."

"But, you know, that's a way they distance themselves," Pauline
said. "It's a defense mechanism because they deal with this kind
of thing all the time. I'm not saying it justifies the harm it does
to the patient, but at least it explains why. And doctors hate
not being able to do anything. They hate feeling impotent. We
see it at the hospital all the time. You know the joke about the
doctor and God?"

"No, tell me."

"Well, a guy dies and he goes up to heaven. There's a huge
long line at the pearly gates so he's told to go and stand at the
end of it. The angel Gabriel says he has to wait his turn so he
gets ready for a long wait. And he waits and he waits and he waits.
The line goes very slowly, and he's getting kind of tired of it.
Then, another little man comes along. He's dressed in a white
coat, with a stethoscope hanging down around his neck. He goes

right straight up to the front of the line. And they let him right into heaven! Well, our man is furious. He yells to the angel, 'Hey, what's going on? Why'd he get to go in right away like that? Who is he?' And the angel answers, 'Oh, don't worry about it. That's God. He likes to play doctor.' "

CHAPTER 6

Commitment

My mother was lucky—she had a lot going for her. She loved life; she loved us kids; and she was crazy about my father. She had always been big on talking, "communicating," even before it became the "in" thing to do. And she was tough—a lot tougher than she thought she was.

That summer Pauline was in a state of shock. She simply couldn't believe what was happening. How *could* it be happening? Everything seemed so normal. David was loving and giving, as usual. He showed no signs of imminent departure. He was strong, as he'd always been, almost as though the disease were an abstract metaphysical thing—a concept rather than a concrete reality. He spoke of it calmly, rationally, almost in the third person. He didn't waver, he didn't panic. To all intents and purposes he was still her rock, as she called him, "my rock, my rock of Gibraltar." He was the one constancy, the one sure thing. Through the years they had seen people splitting up, getting divorced, committing suicide, falling apart all around them. Their union didn't have that element of prerogative. They weren't just tied in a marital contract that could be broken at any time by either party—their union was based on love, blood ties, family. Separation was impossible, at worst it could be only temporary. Could David really die, break that bond, leave her?

It seemed impossible. After all their lunchtime swims, their natural disdain of alcohol and smoking, their health food . . . it was absurd. Absurd, like the recollection of a bad dream that comes back to you as you sip your morning coffee, or warm up the car. But it's not a dream, and you can't understand how the car can start as usual, how the coffee can taste so good.

Pauline was more than just crazy about David. She adored him. "Your father is a genius . . ." she'd say to us, her voice trailing off in amazement. Or: "The way his mind works . . ." Not that that ever kept her from questioning him, or teasing him, occasionally baiting him and refuting him. She loved a good dialogue, a little dialectic. "Your father is not perfect," she'd warn us, as though we could very easily be mistaken on that point. And she'd remind us that he had never cooked a meal in his life although he professed feminism consistently and wanted careers for all us girls. He was a bit out of it—the one time she'd let him go clothes shopping on his own he brought back a pair of pink trousers. He was chronically late, though that had improved significantly since the move to Nashville. And even though he had a photographic memory for scientific data and political facts, one birthday he bought her the same pair of earrings he had given her the previous Hanukkah. "I knew I liked them an awful lot," he said.

Perhaps it would have been easier on Pauline—on all of us— if we had been religious. But we seem to be the kind of family that's more comfortable with unacceptable questions than unacceptable answers. My mother was a critical thinker who looked at everything closely, holding each issue up to the light, turning it to all sides the way she'd examine a dress for stains before buying it. "Who can believe in God after World War II?" she'd ask. And that was that. The bottom line. That one sentence of hers set the tone for religion in our house. David's illness was not about to shake or tempt my mother. It merely confirmed the atheistic tendencies all of us shared. No God would let such a cruel and horrible thing happen. Period. No excuses. No devil, no mysterious ways, no nothing.

Pauline wasn't a cynic. She was a humanist, and she believed in people and their regenerative powers. She herself had an enormous amount of energy, always starting new projects: either planting miniature bonsai trees, doing batiks in the basement, or rearranging the living room furniture. She either loved something or hated it—she was never indifferent. Never blasé. Which made her a great story-teller, because she saw a story, or a point, or even a question, in almost everything she experienced. I remember times she had us on the edge of our seats over a routinely boring faculty meeting. And she had a secret weapon she shared with David: a sense of humor. She believed in laughter almost as much as she didn't believe in God. It was a trick mirror she used on life. If you don't laugh at life, life will laugh at you, goes the old Jewish saying. "Roni," she'd say to me, whenever the subject of men came up, "whatever else you do—get married, don't get married—just make sure the guy has a sense of humor. A sense of humor will get you through anything."

She was always talking to me, telling me things. When I was little she'd call me into the bathroom while she was soaking in the tub. I'd sit on the cold toilet seat and she'd tell me where babies come from, and no, it's not yukky when you love someone. On weekends my sisters and I would crawl into bed with Mom and Dad to talk and giggle. And Mom used to say how each one of us had a different smell, a different feel. Dana was apple blossom herb tea, I was cinnamon and wool and soap, Leora was the smooth bronze sculpture baking in the sun. Michael was too grown up for cuddling by then.

That summer—the first summer of David's illness—was the first time I didn't understand what my mother was telling me, and why. There was an urgency I couldn't place, because the words themselves were dull. Recurrent phrases Pauline used with depth and feeling, to which I could attach only a Webster's definition and no more. Favorite words of hers, like commitment. Trust. Values. Loyalty. "You've got to know what your values are," she'd say. Or: "I don't understand all this open relationship stuff. I trust Daddy. That's what our bond is based on. Trust." She was trying to explain without giving too much away. She was trying to teach me morals without imparting the lessons, tell me conclusions without stories. She was taking short cuts.

The short cuts were taken because my parents decided—at first nonverbally, as in a silent pact, but later with caution and deliberation—that they would not tell "the children" about the illness right away. There would be enough pain later on, they reasoned, why not spare us while at all possible. The illness would wreak havoc in our lives as it was, why not let us enjoy blissful ignorance for the time being? Let us continue our normal lives of school and gossip and midnight movies. There would be time enough later to learn the news, to grieve and adjust. A few months of innocence—what harm could it do? It was not as if we had to seize the time to repair old wounds, to resolve rifts. We had always been a family that shared everything and loved fully. We had no debts to pay, no accounts to settle. There was no urgency to seize valuable time. It may seem ironic, but precisely because we had shared so much, Mom and Dad felt we did not have to share this—at least not now, not right away. Because they had always told us everything, been honest and held nothing back, they could afford to hold this back, to be dishonest for once.

For Pauline it was a gut reaction, an instinctual response. Dad supplied the reason behind it, the rationale. That was the way they worked things out: she feeling the issues, he weighing them. Mom had good instincts, and lots of them. Dad's mind worked like a computer, precise and faster than the speed of light. He could write a treatise on why he took one action or another; she just knew. But she knew without a doubt, and she was rarely wrong.

With us children Pauline was like a mother bear. The mother bear looks harmless playing with her cubs, but don't let that fool you—if you come near those kids, she'll attack. She may appear completely wrapped up in them and unaware, but she's always on alert, all five senses pricked up and ready to go. The least intrusion, the smallest threat—and she'll jump. She'll snarl. She'll put herself on the line.

My mother's first instinct that summer was to protect. To put herself between the terror and the kids. She would guard her cubs. We would be spared.

CHAPTER 7

Gotta Keep Moving

In the "olden days" doctors blamed ALS on a mysterious virus. A virus, they reasoned, invades the body and attacks the nerve cells. But, Dr. Fields had explained to David, this theory had too many holes in it and was soon abandoned. Viruses are infectious; ALS is not. A virus proceeds up to a certain point and then is arrested; ALS is progressive. A virus will usually leave behind remnants or particles which can be identified later in the course of a postmortem biopsy; no such particles have been found in ALS patients.

But another type of virus exists—a virus that acts differently from the average virus, a slow-acting virus that is very difficult both to isolate and to transmit. Kuru, a neurological illness that causes brain damage and is very common among cannibals in New Guinea, is spread by such a virus. The kuru virus must literally be ingested. Usually the disease is not considered contagious, but scientists investigating it discovered that this tribe had a unique way of transmitting kuru: one of their rituals involved eating the brains of a recently deceased relative. When the tribe was educated and the practice stopped, the disease disappeared. Research on this slow-acting virus might provide some leads into the cause of ALS.

A corollary of the viral theory is the autoimmune theory. According to this theory, the virus itself is not directly responsible for ALS, but rather, the disease results from the reaction of the immune system long after the initial viral attack has subsided. When a virus attacks the nervous system, the "casualties"— remnants of the nerve cells or tissues it damaged—remain in the bloodstream. The patient's immune system, never having been exposed to these cells floating around before, reacts as though they were foreign and dangerous. It starts making antibodies and setting out to destroy them with a passion. But the antibodies can't differentiate between the healthy nerve cells and the floating casualties, and they proceed with a vicious attack on all the nerves in the body. Ironically, the body's protection system ends up destroying the body.

Several neurologic diseases may have their origins in a disorder of the immune system. In myasthenia gravis, the nerve doesn't communicate its message to the muscle because the intermediary chemical messenger doesn't function properly. Normally, acetylcholine, the chemical messenger, is recognized by a receptor that sits on the muscle. But in myasthenia gravis, a circulating antibody to the receptor attaches itself to the receptor, thereby blocking the pathway so the acetylcholine can't get the message from the nerve through to the muscle. The result is fluctuating weakness and paralysis. The same thing happens in Guillain-Barré Syndrome. A certain amount of nerve fiber breaks down after a viral attack, or after the introduction of a virus through a preventive vaccine (like the swine flu vaccine). The fibers are released into the bloodstream, and the immune system makes antibodies to them. Plasmapheresis therapy, which removes the patient's plasma and replaces it with healthy blood, has managed to cure Guillain-Barré Syndrome. The theory is that plasmapheresis removes all of the circulating antibodies along with the blood. Several doctors have tried treating ALS with plasmapheresis, and that was one of the studies David had asked Fitzgerald to look up for him.

A third theory suggests that toxic wastes or heavy metal residues may precipitate the disease. Lead is known to accumulate in the nervous system, and some people with lead poisoning exhibit ALS-like symptoms. But studies of randomly chosen ALS patients have presented no uniform abnormalities in measured levels of lead or other toxic substances such as mercury or aluminum. Moreover, ALS strikes at random. If an environmental factor were the primary cause of the illness, whole communities would be affected. No such communities exist. So, although environmental conditions may provide the initial insult to which the body responds, the response and the disease itself must be caused by highly individualized factors.

A fourth theory suggests that metabolic factors cause ALS. In order for the cells to grow and behave normally, their environment must be normal. With this in mind, scientists have measured levels of various substances in ALS patients and compared the data with those of a healthy control group. Sometimes variations are recorded, but it is hard to tell whether they are causes or effects of the illness. Potassium, for example, is abnormally low in ALS patients, but this is probably an effect rather than a cause of muscle wasting.

But all these were theories. A theory can't offer a cure, a treatment, a way out—which was what David was seeking. Still, he felt intuitively that if he stayed in shape the extent of deterioration from the illness would be limited. Not that being out of shape precipitates illness. But David genuinely believed that if he swam, exercised, and ate lots of protein and fresh vegetables, his body would continue functioning. There was a theory behind this modality. David's approach was physiological. Under normal circumstances, muscle will grow if you exercise it. It needs certain things, like a constant blood supply, the right hormones, and good nutrition. But, within that context, physical exercise is still terribly important. Without it "disuse atrophy" occurs—the kind of wasting of muscle that takes place when a limb is in a cast. Why not apply the same principles to diseased muscle? Exercise it and it will grow. That was a universally accepted rule in the medical world. There was only one exception you had to make, and that had to do with fatigue. Fatigue is permissible in healthy muscle, but sick muscle can be so weakened by it that it will never recover. All of the ALS literature stressed that fatigue had to be avoided at all costs. It was printed in all the pamphlets, reiterated by the experts. David decided to exercise regularly— but always stopping short of fatigue.

Swimming would be his primary focus, because swimming exercises just about all of the muscles in the body, especially the respiratory muscles. For his legs David would ride a stationary bicycle; for his arms, wrists, and elbows he would lift weights. For the swallowing muscles he bought himself hard candy, because when you suck on hard candy you're constantly swallowing the saliva you make. All of these ideas were controversial. They weren't endorsed by any of David's doctors. One of the pamphlets from a prominent clinic about ALS said that "an exercise program selected by the physician can be helpful in strengthening unaffected or less affected muscles." But all of David's muscles were affected. So where did that leave him? The pamphlet also said, "Calisthenics serve no useful purpose and may fatigue muscles unnecessarily." David knew that he didn't want to shorten his life by being a hero—or a martyr. He believed in moderation and had no intention of pushing himself too far and driving his muscles to death. But he desperately needed some encouragement. So far, Pauline had been his only source of support. He went swimming, but every time he pulled himself out of the water he thought: "I must be crazy to be doing this. What am I doing? This is utterly foolish."

Towards the end of July, something very important happened. David got home from work to find a very large envelope had been slid under the door. Inside it was an article about plasmapheresis by Dr. Ralph Brewster. Attached to it was a small piece of paper with Brewster's address and phone number. Fitzgerald was no optimist, but he at least got things done.

David called Dr. Brewster that evening. No, he wasn't treating ALS patients with plasmapheresis anymore. Those experiments were three years old, and since then the results had not been very encouraging.

"But, hey," Brewster asked, "are you swimming?"

"Yes, I am, actually."

"Terrific! Keep it up. It's very therapeutic. How much are you swimming?"

"About three-quarters of a mile to a mile every day."

"Good, it's important to do it every day."

"I do, I do."

"Okay, work your way up to a mile and a half or even two. Do you have your own pool?"

"No, I've been going to the Y and the university pool."

"Well, build yourself a pool in the back yard. You should have it right next to you. It's going to get harder to get around and you'll have less energy and you won't be as motivated. Especially in the winter, you'll find all kinds of excuses not to go out—so put it in your yard and throw a bubble over it in the winter, that way it's right under your nose. What other exercises are you doing?"

"I've got a stationary bicycle and some dumbbell weights that I lift and some little gadgets for my hands and my fingers."

"Sounds like you're in great shape. Whatever else you do, stay active. The people who live longest with this disease are the ones who stay active. Listen, you're a doctor and you know what the prognosis is. But I've got three or four patients who have stabilized. I'm not saying they're back to normal, because they aren't, but I've got one patient who was diagnosed twelve years ago and he's still going strong."

"That reminds me of another thing I wanted to ask you, Dr. Brewster. I was planning a trip to South Africa to give some lectures and to see my family, who live there, especially my mother. It's a long trip, but my son will be with me and right now I'm still mobile. I've just got foot-drop in my left leg. Do you think it's a bad idea to go?"

"Hell, no. Go! Why not? Just don't tire yourself—don't run around that much, just do what you have to do, and make sure to rest and keep up your swimming. Right now, you're fit and well, there's no reason not to go. On the contrary. Next year, you may not be able to. I'd say go. It'll give you a lift, a psychological boost and that's important when you're tackling this kind of illness. Yes—I'd say go."

CHAPTER 8

A Fighting Chance

The conversation with Brewster marked a crucial turning point in the way David approached his illness. Up until now his doctors had shrugged their shoulders and lowered their eyes. They had made their diagnosis, no treatment existed for this malady, their job was complete and they washed their hands of him. The message implicit in their actions was: Go home, get your papers in order, get ready to die. Brewster was different. He talked to David, not at David. He was warmer over the phone than either Fitzgerald or Fields had been in person. And he gave David an option. For the first time the disease was not presented as all-encompassing, horrible, and omnipotent. It was just a disease after all; someday there would be a cure for it. And it might slow down. Or go into remission. You never know—so hope for the best. Most importantly: you don't have to be a passive observer of your own destruction. You can be active and fight the illness. Exercise. Keep your muscles functioning. *There is a chance.*

For the first time David felt encouraged. It was time to snap out of this depression—enough was enough. The "Why us?", "Why this?", "Why now?" questions would never be answered. He had never believed in a God, certainly not in a personalized God, an archangel sitting on your shoulder measuring sins and deciding destinies, a God that decided that his children's father should die rather than someone else. No, it was just the way the dice had been rolled, the way the cookie crumbled, the ball bounced. The situation was determined; now his job was to find the best way to live with it. Pauline had told him about a psychiatrist who specialized in treating cancer patients. His approach was similar. "Do you want to live?" he'd ask his patients. "If so, I can help you. If you don't, I can't help you. You have cancer. I'm sorry that you have cancer, but that's a fact, an immutable fact. Let's go from there. There's no turning back. Let's see what we can do to make your life as happy and as comfortable as possible."

This attitude paved the way for David's exercise program. He no longer felt he was following a homemade recipe consisting of a little common sense, a little intuition, and a lot of false hope. He had professional support from a renowned neurologist who conducted pioneering research in the field of ALS. So he piled up a stock of little gadgets to strengthen the muscle of the hands, fingers, and wrists. There was a plastic ball that he could squeeze, a gyroscope Michael had used in swim training, and a "flexer"— a funny contraption that could be used to strengthen the flexor muscles of the hands. Around the house these things were known as "machines" and they were in constant demand.

"Have you seen my machine anywhere?" Dad would ask, a hundred times a day.

"Gosh, I know I saw the black ball machine, but I dunno about the flex machine . . . wasn't it in the car? Hey, Leora, did you bring Dad's machine in from the car?"

"No, but I think I know where it is," Leora would answer, sliding her hand between some cushions or opening a kitchen drawer to pull out a machine or two. She seemed to have a knack for finding them.

In retrospect it's hard to believe: We didn't suspect a thing. I am ashamed to say it, a sure indictment of selfishness and self-involvement. But it was a hectic summer. Mike and David weren't the only ones coming and going. Leora was busy with tennis lessons and Dana went off to a music camp. I was working part-time and off to the woods any chance I had. There were out-of-town guests as well: friends of mine from college, David and Pauline's old friends from Baltimore. Other weekends David was off doing the lecture circuit. As we ran in and out, catching glimpses of one another, subtleties were lost on us. When someone becomes acutely ill he misses work, goes to the hospital, looks awful, and stays in bed. Dad was doing none of these. We weren't about to go out of our way to hypothesize that he had a terminal illness. There was, in essence, no evidence whatsoever. Why exercise the hands? The doctor said so, he said all the muscles should be kept in shape. Just common sense.

A stranger off the street would have seen the unusual in this but we didn't. In our eyes David was impregnable. He was incapable of weakness. If Pauline had been exercising her hands and limping, we would have guessed. We would have known immediately. She was vulnerable. Her health had always fluctuated, so with her, illness was always a possibility. But David was the last person in the world I would have imagined ill. I had never seen him ill. I had never seen him in bed with a fever, a cold, nothing. I'd never seen him sweat or shiver. Never heard him sneeze. The only time he cleared his throat was during a lecture. I had never seen him with a thermometer in his mouth. Or taking aspirin. Or chewing vitamin C. I had never brought him hot tea in bed. He never had to diet to keep his weight down. Never had high blood pressure. David's body was a perfectly functioning machine that needed no special care or attention. It just ran on its own. So now, after all these years, there was a kink in the system. But it was a slipped disk—a superficial kink, just a mechanical error. The thought that it could be thorough, comprehensive, all-encompassing; an organic malfunction, a disease rather than a disorder—never occurred to any of us that summer. Anyway, I myself was so busy being amazed at how wonderfully Dad was coping with the slight malfunction that I couldn't even imagine it was worse than he said. I thought he was a saint because he never complained, never cursed or became impatient, never snapped at us. He just acted normal. And he was so disciplined about his exercise, following the doctor's orders like the perfect patient.

Swimming became a part of the daily routine. Pauline usually accompanied David, if not during their lunch hour, then in the evening. They'd eat dinner, watch the news, then go for a swim. They considered building a pool as Brewster had suggested, and toyed with the idea of putting it in the basement so we could use it year round. But our next-door neighbor had a pool in her yard, which she said we could use "whenever." In the winter

David could join one of the indoor pools in town—at the Jewish Community Center or the Y. Right now he could still drive and get around reasonably well on his own. Next winter . . . he'd just wait and see.

It was tempting to take a Pollyanna attitude to the future, especially after talking to Brewster, but David was aware of the dangers in such an attitude. Perhaps he could not have done it anyway, because as a physician he knew the realities of the illness so well. He knew that the worst was yet to come, that at any stage the worst was yet to come. That's what he found so frightening about the illness. At any given stage, *you ain't seen nothin' yet.* Preparations had to be made for the future. Hope was essential, but it had to be tempered with realism.

Up until now David had been preparing himself negatively. The rabbi and the music. Trivial really. There were more important issues at stake. Family finances, for one. The family should be in as little debt as possible. They were considering trading in the old station wagon for a new car but that could be postponed for a while. All of their papers were in order—his lawyer had always been strict about that. Lucky. He didn't think he'd have the energy to fool with it himself. And they had reasonable insurance policies—also the lawyer's advice. He might be eligible for some additional policies, but he doubted it. Not with this disease. Or else, at outrageous premiums.

There were so many things David still wanted to do. He wanted to get started on the male contraceptive research and he wanted to finish the endocrinology textbook he was co-authoring with a colleague. The book would be a legacy, a record of his clinical experience of the past twenty-five years. Something to leave behind. The NIH had funded him all those years; this was a way to repay the debt. And he wanted to train some younger physicians to take over . . . he didn't want the division at Vanderbilt to fall apart when he left. He wanted to see me graduate from college. And Pauline receive tenure at Vanderbilt. And damn it, he wanted to see Dana and Leora through high school.

Most important of all was a more general question. How was he going to live out his remaining life? He wanted to get the most out of the time he had left, and that meant enjoying every day. Enjoying his work and his family. Enjoying music and theater. Laughing, and making other people laugh. Helping his kids plan for the future. Discussing politics, and mulling over the *New York Times* on a Sunday afternoon. Why should any of that change? It had meant a lot to him before, when he thought that he would live forever. What was the difference now? Everyone had a ticket; the only difference was that his had a date on it.

In retrospect he grew angrier at his doctors. They had done nothing for him, and he resented the nihilistic attitude they conveyed, their cold manner and detachment. He remembered an interview with a muscular dystrophy patient. The man was asked how he defined humanness. "Humanness," he replied, "means being considered a person, not just someone diseased." But David's doctors had regarded him as nothing more than a diseased body. His illness had transformed him irrevocably in their eyes, had cost him his status as human being. They looked at him and saw only ALS. Creeping paralysis. A goner. Not a husband or a father or a scientist. Or a lover, a doctor, a friend. Fields had taken notes from the very first second of their first interview! Not that that was bad on its own—he took notes himself when talking to a patient. But only after he'd put the patient at ease. He wanted to get a picture of the person's situation first, not simply view him as a clinical curiosity. How much knowledge can the patient cope with at the present time? Is the spouse supportive? Is there stress at home? Can he or she miss a few days of work for treatment, or is that out of the question? And David had been dealing with infertility problems, not terminal illness.

Perhaps he was naive. Perhaps he should not have been so surprised. He had always been concerned about the doctor's loss of humanity. It had come up often in conversations with Pauline. She complained that medical students didn't take psychiatry seriously enough. That they didn't appreciate the role mental attitude played in physical illness. That this stance was encouraged by the universities, which select students on the basis of impersonal scores and numbers, and also nurtured by the trend toward superspecialization.

Still. "Primum Non Nocere." The essence of the physician's oath: Above all, do no harm. Doesn't psychological harm count? How many times had he heard the phrase, "He just got so depressed when he heard the diagnosis that he withered away in three months"? Didn't a lot depend upon how the diagnosis had been presented? Would that have happened to him if he hadn't spoken to Brewster?

It was a moot question. The disease obviously had drastically different courses of progression from individual to individual. The point was that an alternative way of handling this illness existed. A way that was guided by hope. All an ill patient needs to hear is that nine out of ten die, and he or she can hope to be that tenth one, the lucky one, the survivor. It's a gamble but it's better than nothing. Hope is an essential ingredient for combating chronic illness. It's an essential ingredient for any life. It's one thing when you're speaking of a finite amount of time, but no doctor can ever determine that. In ALS it can be three months or ten years. Either way is too long to live without hope.

For the first time David understood what it was to be a patient. You feel so vulnerable. You've lost control over your very own body—your environment—your future. The doctor is the only one who appears to have any control at all, so you look to him. Of course, you want a cure, but if that isn't available you'll settle for the next best thing—a modicum of support. Neurologists like Fields, who maintain a strictly technical approach to their profession and disregard the art and "laying on of hands," are of no help in ALS—"no more use to me than the milkman," as one ALS patient wrote. But it doesn't have to be that way. Sure, the duties of a physician embrace diagnosis and treatment. But when that is not available, or no longer effective, they should also embrace continued support of the patient. In his 1858 "Brief Exposition of Rational Medicine," Jacob Bigelow claimed the doctor's responsibility to the incurable patient is "to provide safe passage."* Fitzgerald was doing nothing to provide safe passage for David. If he had just called to check up on him, to make sure he wasn't suicidal. Dropped by, to see how he was adjusting. It seemed only human.

What made Elliot Fitzgerald's absence even more noticeable was that he was the first person in Nashville who was privy to

---

* David and Pauline Rabin expanded this theme in their book, *To Provide Safe Passage*, published in January 1985 by The Philosophical Library.

the diagnosis, and he knew it. David had told him that he didn't want to broadcast the news of his illness because he wanted the family to maintain a normal lifestyle for as long as possible. Of course, it meant he and Pauline had no one to turn to but each the diagnosis, and he knew it. David had told him that he didn't other. Fitzgerald respected their decision, but he made himself scarce.

Actually, there was another person in Nashville who knew the diagnosis: Cheryl Fitzgerald, the doctor's wife. David could pinpoint the exact day on which her husband had told her about his illness because her manner changed abruptly overnight. One day she was pleasant and polite on the phone as usual, and the next day she was curt and impersonal. David had called for Elliot, and when she recognized his voice she couldn't get off the phone fast enough. "Hello-David-how-are-you-we're-all-fine-thank-you-just-a-minute-and-I'll-call-Elliot-he's-right-here-hang-on," she said in one breath, and David heard the receiver drop to the floor as she ran off.

Months later my father relayed this incident to me. He was very philosophical about it. "He shouldn't have told her," he said. "Besides the fact that it was a violation of confidence, she clearly couldn't handle the knowledge. It was a burden to her. Spouses often confide in each other. It's to be expected, I suppose. But they should be more cautious, especially in cases like these. I mean, here was a woman with whom I had chatted amicably at parties, and she couldn't even muster up the courage to say a few words to me. I knew right away she never would again. That any future meeting would be awkward and difficult."

He was right about that. He and Cheryl were rarely in the same place at the same time, but when they were she seemed to avoid his gaze. But David had no idea Cheryl's reaction was a typical one—one he would encounter frequently in the future.

CHAPTER 9

South Africa

In August David boarded a plane to Johannesburg. It had been two months since he'd experienced his first symptoms, one month since the diagnosis of ALS had been confirmed. He was ambivalent about making the trip, and had already decided not to tell the South African part of the family the diagnosis. They had only a few weeks to spend together—why spoil the reunion? And as far as his mother was concerned, she did not have much longer to live; let her go in peace. He would say he had dislocated a disk and leave it at that. Before he left Nashville he promised Pauline that he'd call her every four or five days. She inspected his suitcase and packed in some extra sweaters. It could snow in Jo-burg in August, she said, well, once every ten years or so. Was he going to keep up his exercise? Yes, he assured her, Michael would see to that.

My brother Michael had been swimming competitively since sixth grade. All through high school he got up at five-thirty, when it was still pitch black outside, and rode his bike down to the Y for two hours of swim practice before school. Then after school two more hours. He was in great shape; he had swum all through college and in his senior year he broke the school record for the two-hundred-yard butterfly. He had hard, thickset shoulders and he was very sure of himself—a bit too sure of himself, that summer. "So handsome—and a mensch," the Jewish mothers used to say, wishing him for their daughters, with his sharp blue eyes, and the mop of brown hair over his forehead bleached near blond in the sun.

He kept an eye on Dad that summer. He would watch him move his legs and then try to explain to him which movements he was omitting as he raised his foot off the floor to take a step. Of course, David was leaving those movements out because he was no longer capable of doing them. He had lost those muscles, they simply weren't there anymore. But Michael didn't realize that. And Dad was surprised at how readily Michael accepted the slipped disk explanation, surprised that he didn't suspect something worse. He knew so much about anatomy. Of course there were MD's at the hospital who would believe the disk story for a whole year. You don't see what you don't want to see. And Dad pulled off the life-as-usual stunt terrifically. He was active and gregarious; he joked a lot and made terrible puns that we groaned at, yet repeated to others; he never complained about his difficulties walking and in general made it very easy to forget that anything was wrong. At times he even managed to forget it himself.

Michael saw to it that David swam every day while he was in South Africa. "I think this is the best—the ideal, really—way to approach back trouble," he used to tell David. "And in a way, you know, it's a blessing in disguise. The disk. It's no big deal and you'll get over it but it's a hint. You were running around the country so much. Do you realize how often you've been going away to lecture? Now you have a chance—well, you don't have any choice. You have to pace yourself. Maybe you have to be more selective about the invitations you accept. You have to stay home more and pay attention to your health and diet. Get your priorities straight. So really, it's a blessing in disguise."

That trip was an adventure for Michael. Until then South Africa had existed for us only in newsprint and black and white. Victoria Falls, the Wilds, the big house Mom lived in with the tennis court in front—we had to fill in the colors. Growing up in the United States, we didn't have relatives, we had stories. About Ouma, our grandmother, a large woman who sat in the kitchen at a table laden with figs, chocolate, watermelon, sweet breads, buns. Jack, thirteen years older than Dad, more like a father than a brother to him. A martini every afternoon before dinner, a gold watch for thirty-five years at the firm, a creature of habit. Joyce, the aunt who sends cartons of chocolate to America. Every time she calls she asks what time it is here. "It's always seven hours earlier," we yell into the receiver, but from one call to the next she forgets. "What time is it there now?" she screams across the ocean. We see it merely as an indication of the anachronistic nature of the country itself. Then there is Tots, five years older than Dad, and the spitting image of him. In old photographs of them standing next to each other, I get the impression the picture is a blurred double image. In his youth Tots was the most colorful of them all, a real character, with something to say about everything.

Of the four children David was the youngest—a 1934 "mistake" at the peak of the Depression when all it meant was one more mouth to feed. Ouma and Harry were already deep in debt and they panicked. Harry was a watchmaker. He ran a watch and jewelry store in the little town of Zastron, population eight hundred. He and his father were among thousands of Lithuanian Jews who had left Russia at the turn of the century when a new wave of pogroms broke out. They headed to South Africa on rickety boats, their money tied in bundles and strapped around their waists, to see if it was true what people were saying. Gold on the reef. Gold everywhere. Can't even bury your dog in the backyard without digging it up. Can't even plant yourself a cabbage. If it was true, then Harry's father would return to fetch his wife and the rest of the children. But he never did make it back to Lithuania. He boarded the ship but never arrived. Murdered, his money stolen and body thrown overboard; no one ever found out for sure. Harry was left on the streets of Johannesburg, thirteen years old and unable to speak English. When he used up the money his father had left him, which wasn't much, he took to stealing fruit from street vendors. "Thief!" they yelled after him, a new English word. Finally he managed to apprentice himself to a jeweler. The position gave him a roof over his head, three warm meals a day, and a skill. Learn a trade, he would always tell his children.

Harry was proud and obstinate. When David was born the other shopkeepers were declaring bankruptcy but Harry was still paying back his creditors. He was not going to "lose his name."

It was the biggest mistake he ever made, Dad used to say, since Harry had to sacrifice so much to pay back every penny of his debts. But if you declared bankruptcy you could never open another business under your own name, and that was a disgrace Harry Rabinowitz wouldn't tolerate. Things got worse before the outbreak of World War II when the Afrikaners, caught up in the anti-Semitism flamed by Hitler, joined vigilante "Blackshirts" groups. They bullied Jews in small towns like Zastron, and boycotted their businesses. Those were the good old days when the whites in South Africa could still afford to fight among themselves—a luxury they no longer indulge in. The Jews moved away, on to the next small town, but Harry stayed. He wasn't moving until he'd paid off all his debts. Sometimes it meant that the kids went without food, but by 1940 he was in the clear. The triumph took its toll, however. Harry had changed. He became evry quiet and had a perpetual look of worry and harassment on his face. The family moved that year to Aliwal North.

It was several years later that the family began noticing Harry's strange behavior. He would forget things. He'd be on his way somewhere and he'd forget where he was headed. He couldn't remember where he'd laid down his tools or his book, and he complained of weakness. The town doctor came to examine him. "Your teeth are bad," he said, and pulled them out. All thirty-two of them. But the symptoms persisted. Then Harry said that his eyes were bothering him, and once an avid reader, he now seldom opened a book.

Books didn't mean much in Aliwal North. It was the kind of small town where parents, at the end of the school year, boasted that their children had passed "without opening a book all year." Children used to shove their homework under the sofa if friends stopped in while they were studying. David was an anomaly. He was one of the best rugby players on the high school team, but he read Shakespeare and Milton and scored highest in the province on a national history exam. He was awarded the prize for "Best Chemistry Student in South Africa." Harry was so proud he rustled up enough money to send David on a vacation at the seaside. It was the first time David had seen the ocean. He spent the rest of the summer at a Jewish Habonim camp where he won second place in the debating contests. Harry raved about his son when he returned. He stopped people in the street to boast. Sometimes complete strangers.

But no one said anything about Harry's strange behavior. "Oh Harry?—he's always been like that. Forgetful, that's all it is." Ouma thought that if you didn't talk about it, it would go away. She attributed his illness to moods, quirks. Then one day he couldn't see for three hours. They decided to consult a specialist in Johannesburg. It turned out that Harry had a malignant brain tumor. A vicious kind, an astrocytoma. It was 1950, and chemotherapy hadn't been invented yet. The surgeons had no choice but to operate, even though they knew there wasn't a chance. Astrocytomas don't grow on the linings of the brain like most tumors; they grow right inside the brain. *But no one said anything.*

David was staying with his Aunt Gertie while his parents were away. Gertie was Ouma's sister, an opinionated woman who talked straight. Ouma kept calling, saying everything was fine. Even on the day of the operation: everything's fine. The next day she left a message. David was to come to Jo-burg on the next train. Luckily Gertie was there. She told David his father was sick, much sicker than they had thought; maybe he'd recover but it'd be a miracle if he did, a miracle. David didn't believe in miracles, and on the twenty-four-hour train ride into the capital he realized what Gertie meant. When the train stopped in Bloemfontein, where David's sister Joyce and her husband Sonny lived, and neither was at the platform to greet him, he knew that they must be in Jo-burg already. A few hours later when the conductor came by to punch their tickets and asked for a David Rabinowitz, David said, "That's me." The conductor handed him a telegram, but he didn't even have to read it. He already knew what it said. His father was dead.

Jack and Sonny picked David up at the station. They drove straight to the cemetery. The funeral had already been delayed as long as possible; they were just waiting for David to arrive. All the way there in the car no one said anything.

Back in Johannesburg, David couldn't help remembering all these things. The trip with Michael had been sweet and bitter, point-counterpoint. David had never been one for yarzheit candles, the memorial candles lit on the anniversary of a death, but he carried his father inside him: proud and stubborn, exhorting him to learn a trade, hold your name high. When does shielding your children stop and harming them begin? His own mother's blindness and conspiracy of silence had backfired. They should have gotten Harry to a surgeon earlier. Maybe that was why Ouma had mourned the way she did: no movies, no radio, no music, no tea parties, no nothing for a year and a half. And furious at David's rugby games and cup championships his senior year in high school. Twenty-five years later when Sonny died Joyce did the same thing. Punished herself for surviving. Cut herself off. And Pauline—yes, they had to talk about it. You can't learn from the past if you don't say anything. Shiva, the customary Jewish week of mourning, was cathartic. Two years was excessive, punitive. Life goes on. You cannot stop living after the death of a spouse.

Joyce wanted to remarry now. It had been four years since Sonny had died when she renewed her friendship with an old high school boyfriend, himself a widower. They were already planning the wedding but she was scared to tell Ouma, so she asked David to break the news. David told Ouma after tea one day. Stone silence. "What's wrong?" he asked.

"I never said anything," she protested.

"But you don't have to. It's written all over your face. Joyce is young," David argued, "she's mourned Sonny long enough. She's happy with Abe, and she hasn't really been happy in four years."

"He let her down twenty-five years ago," Ouma replied.

Aha. "But it's not twenty-five years ago now."

Ouma gave in. She couldn't say no to her son. She spoiled him that summer: steak dinners, breakfast in bed. He was a real star now. Oh, he'd always written to tell her about the societies and the honoraria, but what were the Young Turks or the Old Turks to her? Here he was, teaching at Witwatersrand University, and the Lawrence boys said he was the best speaker they'd ever had, and Masie Cohn's girl raved about him . . . now that was nachas, good fortune. David didn't know whether to laugh or to cry, so he laughed. Jack in his quiet, thoughtful way, procured a stationary bicycle for David. Everyone was delighted to meet Michael and take him to Cape Town, to the gold mines, to the game reserve. Joyce was the only one of David's siblings who seemed to know that something was really wrong. Once or twice he caught her looking at him with her eyes scrunched up as though she were staring into the sun. It was the same look he had seen on Leora's face: something's up. So much love.

On the surface, of course, it looked great. He was a celebrity. He enjoyed teaching the endocrinology course at Wits. The students were young, straight from high school, but bright and sharp. They were impressed by this man who talked about dwarfs and insulin from his own experience: he wasn't just relaying to them what he'd read in textbooks—he had seen them, he had studied them. After class they milled around the podium asking him questions. They even sent a committee to their professor to convince him to invite Dr. Rabin back for the following year.

Later David addressed his old professors and classmates at Grand Rounds. He talked about the importance of combining research and clinical practice. He had left South Africa for numerous reasons, he told them, but he had always been loyal to his alma mater for the excellent education it had given him.

It was a difficult speech to give. Looking around the auditorium at the old familiar faces he wondered why he had ever left South Africa. He wanted to climb back into the familiar womb of family and memories and security. At the end of the lecture, professors who had studied with him in medical school came up and clapped him on the back. "Nice job, old chap." "Sorry to see you schlepping a foos." Why had he left?

Of course he knew. He knew only too well.

Most white South Africans are able to justify apartheid because they don't have to look it in the eye day in and day out. As medical students, David and Pauline didn't have that option. The medical class of '56 received its practical training in two hospitals situated across the street from one another: the European Hospital (for whites) and the Non-European Hospital (for blacks). The patients in the white hospital had angina, diabetes, cardiovascular disease and coronary-artery disease. The diseases of affluence and excess—too much sugar, too much cholesterol, fatty foods. Steaks, sour cream, butter, and eggs. Across the street patients were presented with kwashiorkor, scurvy, pellagra, beriberi—the diseases of poverty and neglect. Protein deficiency, vitamin deficiency, not getting enough fresh vegetables. Bloated bellies from hunger and starvation. Here, in the midst of plenty—in "God's own country" as it was so often called, the cornucopia which exported and still exports food—was a dividing line, a street separating black and white. Medicine could not cure many of its ills without radical social and economic change. After all, if a child came in to the hospital with a bloated belly what could the doctor do for him? Admit him, put him on a high protein diet for a few days and pack him on home. But soon he would be back on his previous diet, and return to the hospital within a few months. Health and politics, David and Pauline realized, were inseparable issues. They wondered whether they could remain in the country and tolerate its attitudes while practicing their profession.

During his first year of medical school David didn't think about these issues—the only thing on his mind was excelling in school. He finished the year with three "firsts," and that summer went to work as a counselor at a Jewish day camp for disabled children. The camp had recruited several medical students, one of whom was Pauline. They knew each other by sight, but Pauline was one of the slick city kids who intimidated David, and David, as far as she was concerned, was too smart for his own good. They had been introduced under duress after Pauline had scored a forty-six percent on the physics mid-term. "This is David Rabinowitz," a mutual friend said as he introduced them. "Perfect score again, right, Rab?" Pauline had smiled, nodded, and turned on her heel. Smart-ass! He watched her. Tiny little thing, carrying a huge leather briefcase. She was pretty cute. Nice smile, big white teeth.

They ended up spending the whole summer together. Picnics in the woods surrounding the camp, swimming parties at night with the other counselors. Then, in the fall, tennis at Pauline's house, walks in the garden, Somerset Maugham stories read aloud by the fire. Pauline's father always talking about Zionism—the young Jewish state, and the brave pioneers paving roads, drying swamps, working the land. Double-dating with Pauline's friend Lorraine Cohen and her fiancé, Godfrey Getz. David and Pauline worked on the campus newsletter, typing, writing, interviewing, photocopying, and peddling the paper. In his third year in medical school David was senior editor; Pauline did headlines, editing, and layout. During the fourth year they talked about spending a year in England for further studies after they graduated. Settling in Israel was also a possibility. The medical program was a six-year commitment and they wanted to wait, but they already knew they were going to get married.

In 1956 David and Pauline graduated, David with "First Class Honors." A month later he and Pauline were married. They did their residency training at Baragwanath, a black hospital on the outskirts of Johannesburg, in the area known today as Soweto. A year later Michael Zvi was born, small but healthy. When he was a year old they left for England as planned. They packed two trunks full of clothes. And were deliberately vague when relatives asked if they'd be back in a year's time or not.

The truth was, they really didn't know. They were young and restless, and they were disillusioned with South Africa. They thought of going to Israel or maybe even America—the land of opportunity. It was difficult to leave family and friends, but they knew it would be easier now than later. They hadn't bought a home yet; they were young and made friends easily. They could take their profession with them wherever they went. Leaving the family was tough. But together, they felt, they could do anything. The world was wide open to them.

CHAPTER 10

Normal Living

By Labor Day weekend Michael and David were back from South Africa. The return flight was terrible, Dad said, seventeen hours of night and a horror movie.

That's gross, showing a horror movie on a plane, Leora said.

But just think, it probably helped people who have real fear of flying, Dana suggested.

Stupid, if you ask me, I said.

That was our family: everyone had something to say—on just about everything. It may seem strange, therefore, that my parents kept their secret for as long as they did—almost an entire year. But even more important than sharing their feelings with us was their conviction that we be allowed to go along with our normal lives for as long as possible. "Normal living." It was David's theme, and to a certain extent, his shield. His illness was like the tree that fell in the forest—less real because no one had heard. Because no one knew, it had no consequences. Normal living was proof of that.

That September we had only a few weeks together before scattering to our different corners of the world. I would be going back to Oberlin, Michael would be starting his new job in Chicago, Dana and Leora would be back in high school in Nashville. But those few weeks at the beginning of September, three months after the first terrible morning, set the tone we were to follow for the next few years. Normal living all the way.

There were some behind-the-scenes maneuvers we were unaware of. Mom was not entirely comfortable with the idea of
not telling us about the illness. Particularly in the case of Michael.
Michael was going back up to Chicago at the end of September.
He'd been accepted to the MBA program at Harvard starting in
1981. It was what they called a "deferred admission"—Harvard
likes their young college graduates to get two years of work
experience before starting business school. So Michael had applied
for a job as a computer programs analyst with a utility company
in Chicago. He was to start the first of October. He had looked
for something in Nashville but business opportunities were limited.
Pauline couldn't help thinking: shouldn't they tell him about
David's illness so that he'll stay in town? He was bound to feel
terrible being so far away, and he wouldn't be able to just pack
up and leave in the middle of the job if things got worse. He
should at least have the choice.

David disagreed. Vehemently. Telling Michael wouldn't give
him a choice. On the contrary, it would take the choice away. He'd
feel obligated to stay in Nashville, even if it meant working a
crummy job. There was no way he'd leave for Chicago if he knew.
No way. David knew him. And he knew Michael wouldn't be
able to leave with the knowledge. This is chronic illness, David
told Pauline, not acute illness. You can change your whole life
for a couple of weeks or a month. But for this, you can't. You
have to keep the changes as minimal as possible if you want to
live a halfway decent life. And he was determined not to let this
illness interfere with Michael's career—or for that matter, with
my education, or Dana and Leora's schooling.

There was a risk involved. Michael could end up feeling guilty
later on. Feel bad he hadn't been around to help out. On the
other hand, if he stayed he might feel cheated. Resentful. Lonely.
He didn't know many people in Nashville; the family had moved
here when he started college. He might hold it against them.

Best let sleeping dogs lie. Let him go. Either way it was a
gamble.

Michael and I are opposites. And back then we bounced off
each other, becoming even more extreme. I hated courses, tracks,
anything straight and possibly narrow. I didn't really even want

to go back to school. A friend of mine was going to Alaska to make some money, buy a plot of land. I toyed with the idea of going with him. I also considered going back to Israel and getting another perspective on the country where the family had lived for five years. I had spent my sophomore year of college studying dance, theater, Women's Studies, the Middle East. Health foods, poetry magazines, Pro-Choice. I shouldn't go back to Oberlin until I have some direction, I kept telling myself, but I didn't dare bring it up with the folks. I knew what they'd say: find a direction, kick yourself in the pants. Alaska and Israel will be there in two years. The way tuition's increasing every year we just won't be able to send you to Oberlin two years from now.

There was something else there too. Something they weren't saying and I knew not to ask. Something I sensed in the way Mom cleaned the house, worked in the garden, straightened the fruit in the bowl so it was symmetrical. Everything had to be just right. And we didn't fight or squabble anymore. Dad's dislocated disk was proof of what he always used to say: Life is too short to fight, life is too short to be unhappy; we should realize how lucky we are, all of us are healthy and we stick together.

There was a silence I couldn't pin down. I thought it must be my imagination. Dad and I would sit and have an honest heart-to-heart about my going back to Israel. How it could hurt me, why I should wait to finish my education, how in many ways I am like him, and if I could only learn from his mistakes and be spared his pain . . . but I'd walk away from these talks feeling lonely. Feeling he wasn't confiding in me. That there was a barrier. He'd just told me vulnerable stories but I would feel a detachment, a holding back. Why? I must be crazy, I told myself, and chided myself for being selfish, for expecting more than I ever could have.

I asked my mother to explain one more time. What was a slipped disk exactly? Okay, there's this vertebra and it's pressing down on the nerve. It pinches the nerve and the nerve pinches the leg. Where does the disk come in then? Well, actually it's the disk that pinches the nerve. Well, why don't you say so? What do most people do? Surgery? Well yes, but it's very dangerous—if they cut the nerve, you see. Daddy doesn't really believe it can help.

Her explanation bothered me. What did she mean, "Daddy doesn't believe it can help"? And why didn't she sit down and

draw a little diagram like she did years before when she explained
birth control and menstruation?

I didn't connect this with the floating sensation of unease, and
that feeling of the barrier which must have been my own imagination anyway. It was all so subtle, the ebb and flow of family
life. Non-specific anxiety. Like background radiation. I pre-
registered for psychology, Western Civ, literature courses. And
I packed to go back to school.

My sisters must have sensed something too.

Dana and Leora: the contradictory couplet. Dana loves
eighteenth-century novels. She has wavy hair and soft skin, and
she sees things rosy. She has time and patience; things come
around. Her room is pale blue and she collects shells and hour
glasses and things with her name on them. Leora's skinny, an
inch taller. She's sharp, talks straight like Gertie. Got an answer
to everything. One day she went in to buy school supplies at the
drugstore, but after the saleslady rang them up she decided it was
too much money and she'd changed her mind anyway. Ten minutes later she was back in the store to buy gum. "Sure you want
this now?" the saleslady asked. "I'm sorry, what do you mean?"
Leora asked, all innocent. "Oh, excuse me, I must've confused
you with someone else . . ." the saleslady said, apologizing.

Dana sees the good things, exaggerates them. It's a trait she
inherited from her father. Leora's suspicious; she's a digger.
Why is Dad exercising his hands if his legs are hurt, she wanted
to know. Well, the same nerves that the disk catches go to the
arms as well, Mom answered. Oh yeah, Leora said.

Normal living. It meant understanding all about Dad's research
on the male contraceptive. It meant running to the store in the
middle of the night to satisfy cravings for chocolate or Pepperidge
Farm cookies. Most of all, in our household, it meant eating
dinner together. Dinner was a big deal. It wasn't formal—
usually thrown together at the last minute, steaks chucked in
the oven and whip up a salad—but the table was always set, and
everyone's presence required. Absolutely no TV or newspapers.
And no skipping. Staying away from dinner was almost a betrayal.
You really had to have a good excuse. Besides, you'd be missing
out on some good fun.

"Which bozo set the table this time?" Michael asked one night, as he noticed there was no salt or pepper or water or salad dressing out.

"We called you to help, hon," I said.

"I don't know why you're sitting down already. Dad isn't here yet," Dana said.

"That's his car in the driveway right now," Mom said, peeking out the window. "He just wanted to swim before dinner because the Bowers are coming over for coffee this evening."

"Great, 'cause I'm starving. All I ate today was carrots," Leora said.

"You're crazy," I told her.

"You forgot the Milky Way," Dana reminded Leora.

Then came the familiar cry, "The king is here!" and Dad swung open the back door into the kitchen.

"Hi king."

"Hi Dad."

"Hi Daddy."

"Good swim?" Mom asked.

"Terrific. Can I do anything for dinner?"

"Yeah. Sit down," Leora suggested.

"Dad," I said, going to the fridge to pull out an experimental olive and cheese dip I'd concocted, "a friend of mine wants to be a subject in the male contraceptive research and I really didn't know what to tell him. Are you still looking for volunteers? You pay them, don't you? But I sort of remembered they had to be a certain age or married or something."

"Well, you're jumping a little ahead of the game since I don't even have the grant yet. But we will be looking for older men, family men probably," David answered.

"I hate to ask this, but what is this gray stuff, Roni?" someone asked.

"Hey. It's cheese and olive dip and it's good, okay? Besides, are you color blind? It's not gray, it's green. Try it. It's good, really," I said.

'David, why don't you explain to the children a little about how the research is going to work. I don't think we've ever really talked about it," Mom said.

"Well," Dad started, "of course this is all in the theory stage right now. But let me give you a bit of history first so you can understand how the whole thing got started. There are two very important hormones everybody has: LH and FSH. They stand for Luteinizing Hormone and Follicle Stimulating Hormone. Both men and women have them. If they don't have them, they don't develop normally and they don't go through puberty. So if you're lacking them you won't menstruate if you're a girl or won't grow hair on your chest if you're a boy. With me so far?"

"Yeah. Go on."

"We'll stop you if we need some help."

"Well, the next question is, why wouldn't these people have them? Now, hormones are released when they get a message from the brain. Essentially the brain says: 'Okay, time to make some LH and FSH,' and that message pushes the glands into action. So one reason people may not be making LH and FSH is if the brain isn't giving them the message."

"But how does the brain give the message? Is it a chemical type thing?"

"As a matter of fact, it is—it's another hormone that's named for what it does: Luteinizing Hormone Releasing Hormone. Otherwise known as LHRH. The two scientists who isolated LHRH in the late sixties got the Nobel Prize for their work. Their names are Schally and Guillemin. And the first thing they rushed off to see when they got it isolated was whether it would work on patients who are lacking the LH and FSH. And it did."

"So what happened?" Leora asked.

"Well, women who had never ovulated or had their periods and thought they would never be able to have children, had a very nice surprise. You can just imagine how it changed their lives.

"Then something very strange happened. A scientist at the University of Pittsburgh, whose name is Dr. Knobil, did some experiments with monkeys. First he gave them regular injections of LHRH and watched their LH and FSH levels increase. Then he tried something different and gave them a constant infusion of LHRH. Of course he expected the LH and FSH to go out of bounds. But instead, they stopped altogether. It was almost as if the brain was saying, 'Cool it. You're confusing me,' and went on strike. It was just too much of a good thing."

"Can't fool Mother Nature, huh," I said.

"Did the same thing happen in people?" Michael asked.

"Yes. Those were the experiments I did in Israel and the exact same thing happened. The brain just turned off, as if it had been bombarded and just wouldn't respond anymore."

"So that's how it works as a contraceptive . . . I was wondering where this conversation was going . . . "

"Well now, one more important thing happened, and that was in 1975, just about when we moved to Nashville. Two other very brilliant scientists, Vale and Rivier, out in California, developed what is called an analogue to LHRH. An analogue is a twin compound—an almost identical twin. It's made artificially and it's almost exactly like the original material except that it often acts differently. Sometimes it's much more powerful than the original material, and sometimes it does the opposite of what the original does. So how does the LHRH twin act? In the test tube, it's one hundred fifty times stronger than the natural material. But—and this is why research is like a detective novel—in animals, it has the opposite effect. It turns the brain and the hormones off. The effect was similar to that of the constant infusion. The brain says: 'Overload. Go away. Just forget it.' Fantastic! And you're right—that's when we first started thinking about using it as a contraceptive instead of as a fertility agent. It could be a female contraceptive or, just as easily, a male contraceptive."

"What about side effects?"

"We don't know yet. But we plan to be very careful and watch our subjects closely. That's really all we can do. We're hoping this drug will have a much more direct and limited effect than the Pill, for example. So we'll watch our subjects and if there's any sign at all of irregularity we'll pull the men off at once. We'll progress stage by stage; if one stage passes without complications we'll go on to another, and so on."

"Why has it taken so long to get some serious research going on a male Pill?" Michael asked.

"Sexism," I answered, unequivocally.

"Actually, it's much more complicated to devise a Pill for men," Dad said. "A woman has only one egg and one cycle at any given time. You can step in and interrupt that cycle at any point. Men's reproductive mechanisms are constant factories working twenty-four hours a day. It's much harder to disrupt sperm production. There is a cycle of sorts, though. It takes about ten weeks to build a sperm."

"Well, you have to admit, all of the research has been directed at women," Mom said.

"That's true," David answered. "But times are changing."

By the time we exhausted the subject we had finished dinner. Now it was tea-time. Tea, like dinner, was also a family ritual, one of the few my parents brought from South Africa with them. The tea was steeped long and strong; only when it was very black was it poured into teacups. Teacups and saucers. Milk, which was always added, was poured into the cups first. Mom swore it tasted better that way. Sugar could be added, but in moderation. You haven't really acquired a taste for tea until you can drink it without sugar.

Tea-time didn't last long that evening because our friends Wayne and Eve Bower were coming over. My parents had not told the Bowers the truth about David's condition, even though Wayne and Eve were their closest friends in Nashville. Why? Their rationale was the same as the one for the family: normal living. And a fear that once the news was out there would be no controlling it. It would spread like wildfire. Not that they didn't trust the Bowers. It wasn't that at all. Just an irrational fear. The Jewish community was small—just a few thousand people. The hospital was located just across the street from Dana and Leora's high school. Even if no one said anything, children pick up on subtleties. Looks of pity, chicken soup calls. But it wasn't really that either. It was something much deeper, much more fundamental. David wasn't ready to open his guts to the world. He wasn't ready to declare himself a terminal case. He wasn't ready to admit defeat, to acknowledge the fight, to say it out loud. He wasn't even ready to say it to himself. He wanted to go on being himself—strong, independent, giving. Just a little bit longer.

As we waited for the Bowers, we discussed Michael's new apartment and how much utilities could cost in the cold Chicago winter, whether Dana and Leora should take a computer course in high school this year and whether one was even offered; if I could get a cheaper flight back to school. Normal living.

But in the next few weeks two things happened that scared the hell out of us. And when they were over, they left us with a strange, but very powerful, illusion of safety and security. And with the feeling that nothing more could possibly go wrong.

Two days before I was to fly off to Oberlin—it must have been the fourteenth or fifteenth of September—Michael had a terrible car accident. He had fallen asleep at the wheel of our big heavy station wagon. When he woke up, his hands were clutching the steering wheel in a tight grip and he was staring a telephone pole in the face. The telephone pole had bashed right through the body of the car and seemed about to break in through the front windshield. The car was motionless—arrested by the impact of the pole—but Michael instinctively put his foot on the brake. Still holding tight to the wheel he tried to remember: how many beers had he had?

Just then a policeman stuck his face in through the window. He stared at Michael for a few seconds, then asked him gently: "You all right, son?"

Michael took a while to respond. He was in a daze, but he was fine, and he opened the door and slowly climbed out of the car. Barely a scratch. Just a little one on his face. Lucky. He had quick reflexes. Athlete's reflexes. Even asleep, he had clutched on to that wheel and held on.

"You're a mighty lucky fellow," the policeman told him. "Mighty lucky. Go to church this Sunday, I tell ya. I just came here from picking up a guy just like you—had a little drink and took himself a nap. Went flying through the windshield and cracked his skull open. I took him straight to the morgue."

When Michael relayed the story to us later on, he repeated what the policeman had said. "I took him straight to the morgue." The significance was lost on no one. Michael had barely made it. It was a narrow escape. Literally, a brush with death. We felt a collective rush of relief, as though we'd just stepped off a roller coaster onto solid ground. Only Mom and Dad knew this was just the beginning of the ride. And they were scared. All it proved to them was that there are no guarantees, no assurances, not even now that they had seen the worst. When they packed me off to Oberlin they loaded me up with advice and precautions that were as heavy as cumbersome baggage. Be careful. Call us when you get in. Don't do anything silly. Don't walk alone at night.

About a week later, just as I was settling into my new place at school, they called with some terrible news: Mom had developed a lump in her breast. They didn't know yet. It could go either way. She had had these things before. She was going into the hospital for a biopsy the next day.

Why did they choose to tell us this, and not the other bad news? Cancer is an outspoken illness: the process of detecting and treating it is noisy. The mere existence of a process of therapy assures that. It could not be hidden even if they had wanted to hide it. And not only that; they simply couldn't hide any more at this stage. There was only so much they could do alone, and they were reaching the limit.

I somehow knew Mom would be okay. I knew the biopsy would be benign. There was no good reason for this feeling, but there it was. I was confident. There was no need to fret: we could always begin fretting later, I told myself. She'd had biopsies before. She had cystic breasts. It wasn't an emergency. Better check it out than leave it be, no doubt. But I was very calm, and very sure.

Mom had no such confidence. Why should she? The "It can't happen to me" shield was long gone, eradicated. Who's to say "It can't happen to both of us"? No one was up there counting, making sure our family received only our due and no more. Anyway, was David's illness our due? Surely not. What had we done to deserve it? Nothing. And what if both she and David were struck with such horrible illnesses? She couldn't even imagine.

Pauline was petrified. But as scared as she was of being ill, she was even more scared of being healthy. She really didn't want a verdict either way. She had a bit of flu and delayed the biopsy. Then she delayed it again, just to put it off. She just couldn't face the truth either way. The thought of carrying on, of living the next day and the next, frightened her. At least if she was sick she could sink back, tea in bed, all taken care of. Stop time. And she had the superstitious certainty that both she and David could not be struck at once: if she was declared ill, he would get better. It had to work that way. The doctors would discover a ghastly error. They had misdiagnosed his condition.

He'd have no choice but to get better. He'd have to be there for her, for the children. He was strong, he could manage without her. But she, without him? It was impossible to imagine, to conceive.

The prospect of her own illness sunk Pauline into total despair. In the late afternoons she would slink off into her room, and doze on her bed to the sounds of Mozart and Bach. On the days preceding the scheduled biopsy David had to coax her out of bed to go to work in the mornings. "You don't realize how lucky you are," she wanted to say to her psychiatric patients, and send them on their way. The eight o'clock one, who wanted to complete his Ph.D" but-why-should-he-just-because-it's-expected-of-him-even-though-he-might-as-well-he's-come-this-far-but-he-can't-make-up-his-mind. "You don't realize—you're both healthy!" to the nine o'clock couple who were in the middle of a messy divorce. She wanted the new car and the cat and of course the kids but he wanted the maid who had been with them for years and the condo with the pool and wall-to-wall carpeting . . . "You don't realize!" she wanted to say. But she didn't. She kept her mouth shut, listened and counseled. She was a professional.

Finally Pauline entered the hospital for the biopsy. David wouldn't let her put it off any longer. The news was good, and there was no question about the diagnosis: the lump was benign. The verdict shook Pauline out of her numbness. She knew that she was well, and that she had a job to do. Once again David had taken care of her. Now it was her turn.

As for the rest of us, we again had that feeling of narrow escape. But now, we thought, everything was going to be okay. Everything was going to be just fine.

CHAPTER 11

"Just a Bad Back"

In October David returned to his normal routine at the hospital. Nothing had changed as far as anyone could tell; Dr. Rabin just had a bit of a disk problem. "Oh boy," his colleagues would say when he told them what was wrong, "Boy, I had a disk once too— let me tell ya . . ." and they would launch into long monologues about swimming, discipline, surgery, the options, the pain. David would nod and put in his two cents' worth; then they would pat him on the back and wish him the best. He was still one of the club. He was still in the right kingdom, as Susan Sontag has said. You know how you stop when someone passes you on the street on crutches? You stop to check them out—temporary mishap or permanent damage? You categorize them in your mind: one of us or one of them? Which passport do they carry—of the ill or of the well? The difference between a dislocated disk and amyotrophic lateral sclerosis is the difference between a broken leg and a cripple. A broken leg only puts you on probation; you still belong. Paraplegics have their passport unconditionally revoked. And in the context of the medical profession it is even more important to be in the right kingdom—the kingdom of the well. In the midst of the healers the sick are not merely aliens, aberrations, nuisances—they are traitors.

On the rare occasions that David bumped into Fitzgerald, the neurologist looked depressed, as if to say: thanks a lot, David, you just ruined my day. He would shift his weight nervously from one leg to another, trying to think of something to say. David came away from these chance meetings feeling dejected and uncomfortable. He would have to sit down for a while, pull himself together, remind himself of the resolutions he'd made and his determination to fight this illness. Fitzgerald probably wouldn't believe it, but David had already seen new muscles develop from the swimming. His favorite stroke, half free-style and half breaststroke, had built up his chest and shoulder muscles enormously. In fact, later on, these muscles would enable him to stay on his feet, supplementing the loss of strength and balance in his legs with his arms and a crutch.

At the end of the month David took a trip to Ireland to meet with Dr. McKenna, the co-author of the endocrinology text. McKenna was alarmed by the deterioration that had taken place in David's walking since June, when they had last seen one another.

"Don't worry," David assured him, "I'm doing everything my doctors told me. All I need is a pool so I can keep my swimming up."

"The outdoor pools are closed already and there's only one indoor pool in Dublin. Last time I was there it wasn't very enticing. Really filthy. You can give it a try. It's not too far from here."

So the next day David walked over to the pool. McKenna was right: it was filthy. The water was a dark shade of green, and the change rooms were wet and moldy. David asked to see the manager.

"Good afternoon," he said. "My name is Dr. David Rabin, I'm from Vanderbilt University in the United States. I've come to Dublin to work with my colleague at the university here. His name is Dr. Joseph McKenna. I'm on a strict exercise program prescribed by my doctors. It can't be interrupted for even the smallest amount of time—unfortunately." He laughed. "Part of it requires swimming. This is the only indoor pool in town, or so Joe tells me. But it's awfully unsanitary and I can't possibly swim in it. It probably constitutes a health hazard. So if you would clean it up I'd be very grateful. I'm going to be here for two weeks and I'll be swimming every day. If you don't, I'll have no choice but to call the Health Department."

McKenna laughed when David told him the story. "Good try,

David, but this isn't America. This is Ireland. It doesn't work that way here. That chap knows that by the time you get through to the Health Department, and by the time the clerk decides what to do with the message, and by the time he passes it on to someone else, and it lies on that chap's desk for a few months . . . why, you'll be long gone out of the country! There's so much red tape here. And tea breaks, and rigamarole. You can't imagine what I go through to get a package from the basement up to my laboratory. Can't go fetch it myself, for the unions. It can take weeks."

But the next day David went back to the pool and found that the brackish water had been replaced with clear blue, and in the dressing rooms the peeling paint had been scraped off and the moldy shower curtains removed. Two young men in overalls were mixing gallon jars of fresh green paint. He changed into his suit and walked out to the pool.

CHAPTER 12

Hope and Lecithin

David flew to Canada to meet Dr. Brewster, the physician who had conducted the plasmapheresis experiments, on November 4, 1979. David had spoken to Brewster by telephone several times and been encouraged by his positive attitude so he decided to go to meet him. He remembered the date because it was the same day that the Americans were taken hostage in Teheran. Imprisoned—a term which had often been applied to describe ALS patients. "Prisoners in their own bodies." Locked in. Minds without an outlet. A sentence to live out.

Traveling was an escape, though. Flying, covering miles. Taxis, airports, traffic, train stations, hustle and bustle. Timing, schedules, deadlines, appointments, meeting places, interviews, action. Doing, talking, theorizing.

His limp was more pronounced now. His left foot drooped so much that unless he raised the hip to a ninety-degree angle his toes would drag on the floor and trip him. He took elevators, never escalators; and he tried to plan for the winter. Naturalists were predicting a harsh one—they'd found more spider webs than usual, and there was something about caterpillars' fur. David's philosophy was that you had to be practical about these things to avoid panic later on, so he bought bags of sand and salt for the driveway, and a down coat. The kids had suggested the latter—it was light but very warm.

In Brewster's offices a strange incident occurred. David was sitting in the reception room filling out little three-by-five cards with his name, address, insurance company and policy number. Name, address, place of employment, age. Name, address, telephone number—

"Are you here to see Dr. Brewster because you have ALS?" a voice intruded on his thoughts.

David looked up from the cards and stared at the receptionist who had asked the question. He was stunned. It took him about thirty seconds to regain his composure.

"That," he then answered, "is between me and my doctor." He said it slowly and deliberately. Then he returned to his cards.

The receptionist glared. Now she would have to wait for another whole hour to get a glimpse of the doctor's notes. But that must be what he had! Just starting off too. He looked all right. Just that funny way of throwing his leg. But why else would he have come all the way from Nashville to see Dr. Brewster? Hideous disease.

A few minutes later a patient left, and a nurse came out to tell David the doctor would see him. She took him into the examining room, and Brewster, who was sitting behind his desk, rose to greet David. He was tall and wiry, with a youthful face and a mop of curly hair. All his movements were quick, brisk, and energetic. He shook David's hands between both of his, and picked up right where the telephone conversation had left off in July. "Did you see that man who just left my office? Walking with a cane?" he asked. David nodded. He had noticed the patient when he came in.

"He's had ALS for fourteen years," Brewster continued. "Unbelievable, huh? He works, takes care of his family, lives a normal life. And I've got other patients like that. Oh, they work at it, work hard every day. Which means spending a good four-five hours in the pool rain or shine. But that man was diagnosed fourteen years ago and he's walking with a cane. I've got another patient I diagnosed twenty years ago—also walking around. Sometimes he uses a walker. He has good days and bad days, like the rest of us, but generally, still active, still getting around."

To David, it sounded almost too good to be true. Those were just two patients—out of a pool of how many? Twenty? Fifty?

A hundred? Realistically speaking, David wondered, what were the odds? David's illness had already reached the stage of the fourteen-year patient—in just five months. He had resisted a cane so far but it would just be a matter of time. And he knew his limits. Four hours in the pool would knock him out. It would have knocked him out before the illness. He liked Brewster's approach. But how reliable was it? Were the ALS patients doing well because they were active, or were they still active because they were doing well? How reliable was this guy?

David's suspicions were confirmed during the physical examination, when Brewster completely missed the weakness that Fields had located. And then the doctor suggested what at first sounded preposterous: that perhaps David had been misdiagnosed. There was a rare form of syphilis which produced ALS-like symptoms, and perhaps that was the cause of David's disability. It was difficult to detect this particular form of syphilis and he'd have to do a spinal tap. He could schedule it for the next day if David would stay in Canada. Of course, it was David's choice.

"Hell, why not? It's just a test, might as well find out," David said. He doubted it though. Pauline and he had been faithfully married for twenty-three years. If he had syphilis it would prove the disease could be transmitted by dirty toilet seats. Still, why not have the test? He had nothing to lose. There was always the chance that he had contracted syphilis by some freak accident, and anything was preferable to ALS.

"Is eight too early for you?" Brewster asked. "We can meet here and I'll drive you over to the hospital."

"Thanks. Eight is fine."

"Oh," Brewster said, as an afterthought, "another thing I've been suggesting to patients is lecithin. They've been using it to treat various neurological illnesses." Lecithin is a phospholipid, a form of fat that contains phosphorus. Part of the lecithin molecule contains choline, and when the lecithin is absorbed the choline splits off. Choline is one of the ingredients that together with acetate form acetylcholine, the chemical messenger that links the electrical messenger of the nerve with that of the muscles at the neuromuscular junction. "Why don't you start out taking, say, a capsule every day. It's easily obtainable nowadays. It's become a health-nut sort of thing. Anyway, try that for a while, and we'll stay in touch about it. And I'll see you tomorrow morning."

"Thank you. You've been very supportive. I appreciate it. I really needed a boost back in July, and you gave it to me. You're an optimist, and they are a scarce resource in neurology, and a very valuable resource. Thanks again."

The next day Brewster took Dad over to the hospital. First he ran a lung function test similar to the one Fields had done. The results showed that David had two hundred percent the normal breathing capacity. "That's great, puts you in the best prognostic category," Brewster said.

Next came the spinal tap. Taps can be tricky. A needle has to be inserted in between the vertebrae in order to extract some of the cerebrospinal fluid and the insertion can be difficult. Cerebrospinal fluid, or CSF, is the liquid that bathes the brain. It goes up and down the spine and acts as a buffer of sorts. Certain cells and proteins, including the syphilis bacteria that Brewster was looking for, are easier to measure in the CSF because they are found in higher concentrations than elsewhere in the body. As David had predicted, however, the results were normal.

After the tap David lay flat on his back for twelve hours. The next day he felt fine, got up and walked around a bit, and asked Brewster if he could go swimming. Brewster said sure. David went back to his hotel, swam a mile and a half, confirmed his booking on the evening flight to Nashville, and went out to catch a bite to eat before going to the airport. Halfway through his steak he felt ill. He started vomiting. Holding a napkin to his mouth he escaped to the bathroom. His head was spinning, and he felt as if his brain were dropping down into his spinal cord. The tap had removed less than ten milliliters of spinal fluid but it felt like a gallon was missing. David pulled himself together enough to pay his bill and wobble out to flag a cab. He had his bags with him, and he told the driver to head straight to the airport. His head was still spinning when he boarded the plane, and by the time he changed flights he was vomiting again. The stewardess who was checking tickets stopped him. "I'm sorry, sir. We can't possibly let you on the plane in your condition."

"My condition?" he echoed. She must have thought he was

drunk. "I'm sick. I'm not intoxicated. I'm genuinely ill. I'm a physician, and I've got to get home so I can recuperate."

The stewardess shook her head, and said she was sorry.

"I've made my reservation," David protested, "and I paid for my ticket in advance. There's absolutely no reason for you to deny me service."

She shook her head again, and said she was sorry, *but*. David realized he had to change his tactics if he didn't want to spend the night at the airport.

"You realize this is a violation of my constitutional rights, don't you?" he asked. "And I can assure you that I'll sue the airline if you don't let me on this plane. What is your name, please?" he asked politely as he pulled a pen out of his breast pocket and prepared to write on his boarding pass.

He was speaking very calmly and the stewardess reevaluated. Well, maybe he wasn't drunk. She inhaled deeply. No alcohol on his breath that she could catch. She didn't want any trouble, so what the hell, she let him pass.

For the next three days David lay flat on his back. Every time he pulled himself up to a forty-five degree angle the nausea and dizziness returned. Pauline was anxious. Had he contracted meningitis? She called Fitzgerald and asked him to come over and take a look at David. He did, and assured them that the reaction was extreme, but within the normal range. David should just lie flat for the rest of the week.

It was the first time Pauline had seen Elliot since the diagnosis had been made and when she walked him to the door he blurted out, "I don't know how familiar you are with this illness, Pauline. I'm sure David wants to spare you. But there are some things you should know. You must know, in fact. One of the tragedies of this particular illness is that it does not produce dementia as multiple sclerosis does, for example. So David will know exactly what's happening to him the entire time. I guess that's really the worst part about the whole thing."

Fitzgerald kept on talking, but Pauline was no longer listening. She couldn't believe what he had just said. "One of the tragedies of this particular illness is that it does not produce dementia. . . ." The tragedies? It was one of the blessings! The only blessing, in fact. It is dementia that is the tragedy. How could anyone think it a misfortune that dementia had been averted? This illness would rob David of everything—walking, running, standing, holding—but it wouldn't touch his mind. Fitzgerald must not have been thinking, Pauline reasoned; he must not have thought the idea through. He, like any physician, had seen the effects of dementia: seen once articulate and clearly thinking adults struggle to hold on to simple pieces of information: what time it is, what city this is, the name of an eldest son or daughter. Pauline had counseled the children of these patients, who described how their parents relayed the same meaningless stories over and over again, how their parents no longer knew to keep themselves clean, how they tied name tags onto them in case they got lost. "One of the tragedies is that it does not produce dementia." Worst of all was that the parents of these children no longer responded to them. They could no longer talk, answer, exchange, love. Sometimes they didn't even know who was nursing them. "I'm taking care of a total stranger," one woman told Pauline.

No, there wasn't much to be thankful for with this illness, but that it doesn't affect the mind is one definite plus, Pauline thought. David's mind—what a treasure! The mind that teased, analyzed, solved problems, designed brilliant experiments, helped the kids with their algebra and chemistry and even English papers, taught them new vocabulary, communicated, shared, absorbed—and would continue doing all that. The mind was safe! Spared! It would enable David to continue his work, to continue being a member of the family, to be her David. It was a blessing. David's mind—was David. It was his talking soul. It was his mind that had first attracted her, his mind that kept her interested, his mind that she was in love with. It was his mind that would provide her with support and love over the months to come. Thanks to his mind he would be able to hear her out, discuss her ideas, and help her cope with the tough times to come. How little the doctor understood . . .

And then Pauline remembered David's own role model, the great endocrinologist Fuller Albright. Albright had a bad case of Parkinson's disease. He shook like a leaf, so much that he couldn't walk and it was hard to understand his speech. But that didn't stop him—his mind was clear, and he continued with his work, seeing patients and teaching. He used to say he could handle just about anything his illness brought upon him. The only thing that upset him was when colleagues became impatient with his speech and gave up on trying to understand him. After several years of illness Albright volunteered for an experimental form of brain surgery that was being used to cure Parkinson's. The surgery was a complete disaster, and instead of curing his physical malady it destroyed his brain. He was left without any intellectual capacity whatsoever. That was the tragedy of Fuller Albright—not the illness, but the surgery that put an end to his wonderful contributions.

Even as David lay in bed now his mind was racing. He had told Pauline about Brewster—"a wonderful man, but I think his optimism interferes with his science"—and about lecithin.

"Oh, that must be the stuff they're using to treat Alzheimer's," Pauline had said. Alzheimer's disease is an illness that produces dementia primarily in elderly people, and, according to some studies, the enzyme responsible for binding the acetate and choline together into the neurotransmitter acetylcholine is deficient in Alzheimer's patients. "And tardive dyskinesia as well. Those studies were pretty interesting." Tardive dyskinesia is a side effect of long-term use of psychiatric drugs such as Haldol. These drugs produce an imbalance between different neurotransmitters, one of which is acetylcholine, and the result is a condition that causes involuntary movements of the tongue and mouth. "In more than half of the patients lecithin treatments made a difference."

"Well," David said, "assuming that the amount of choline in the bloodstream can be increased with regular ingestion of lecithin—that's your first 'if'—and assuming that the choline is then transformed into acetylcholine—that's your second 'if'— then, maybe, once more of the chemical messenger is available it'll be easier to transmit the diminished message from the ALS damaged nerve to the muscle. Your third 'if.' So let's do an experiment."

Pauline agreed. "It's a long shot, but anything's a long shot with this illness. They know so little."

"I'm going to start taking lecithin myself," David said. "The only problem is that choline is just one small component of the lecithin compound. I want to be sure I'm getting a substantial amount of choline. It may mean eating a whole lot of lecithin tablets—not just one or two. I'll sit down with a piece of paper and figure it out exactly. Meanwhile, let's try to find out as much as we can, and then run an experiment. Together. You up for it? Test normal healthy subjects for the first two factors in question. What do you think?"

"As long as we don't have to write a grant!" Pauline laughed— she hated writing grants.

"Writing a grant isn't that bad. There are a few tricks to it, that's all. I'll show you."

But writing a grant was just the beginning. David and Pauline threw themselves into a frenzy.

CHAPTER 13

Becoming the Other

The lecithin project absorbed Pauline and David. There was something therapeutic, soothing, and wonderful about working so hard you didn't have time to think, about occupying your brain so it didn't have time left over to fret, worry, despair.

Actually, it started even before the lecithin project. David was already deeply engrossed in his endocrinology textbook. He was teaching himself to dictate the material, partly because it saved time, but partly in preparation for the possibility his hands might give out before he'd finished the text. Then there was the male contraceptive grant—news of which was due any day, toward the end of December or early 1980. The lecithin project would mean an additional load of work—securing funding, designing the experiment, reading the literature, recruiting the volunteers. And there was a personal complement to this project: he was feeding himself large quantities of choline.

It was no small feat. According to David's calculations, he would have to take in at least one hundred grams of lecithin in order to get thirty grams of choline. And he wanted to get at least that much of the enzyme, if not more. Unfortunately, one capsule of lecithin contains only about 2 grams of lecithin—which meant he had to swallow fifty capsules every day! He would sit down, jiggle about half a bottle of pills into his hand, and pop them in his mouth like popcorn. It couldn't have been much fun, but he was very good about it. The question was, how would he convince the volunteers to do it?

He had an idea. Lecithin also came in a granular form. Maybe we could concoct a lecithin milkshake. Leora and I accepted responsibility for the task. We didn't know what we were getting ourselves into. David ordered several kilos of the stuff. When it arrived on the doorstep we thought someone was playing jokes on us. There, on the back porch, was a barrel as big as a garbage can, full of what looked like sand, right off the beach. The grainy formula proved no easier to get down Dad's throat than the capsules. No matter how much ice cream, crushed pineapple, banana, carob chips, flavored yogurt, or honey we put in the milkshake, the grainy taste still came through. Dad took it like a soldier.

David and Pauline began planning the lecithin experiments immediately. They wrote a grant application requesting Vanderbilt to fund the research. While they waited to hear whether the project would be funded, there were other projects on the academic burner. Pauline had to get on the ball about some long overdue cases she'd wanted to write up—she would be coming up for tenure at Vanderbilt a year or two down the road. She wanted to write a paper about suicidal adolescents: the often overlooked children who are casualties of divorce. And the whole problem of the so-called civil rights of the insane. Pauline felt very strongly about this issue. The law really tied psychiatrists' hands. You could commit a patient involuntarily—without the patient's consent—only if the patient was proven to be suicidal or homicidal. Otherwise you had to wait until the patient decided to sign him or herself in.

"In other words, you're asking an irrational person to make a rational decision," David said.

"Exactly," Pauline said. "It deserves a letter to the editor of a journal or newspaper, don't you think?"

"Why not go for a paper? Build up your curriculum vitae. You've got so much knowledge stored up in you," David encouraged her. "You could research the laws. It wasn't always the way it is now. There's been a swing of the pendulum from no rights at all to this extreme situation. It's high time the medical community examined the issue. By the way, when you get done with that paper, I've got another idea for you."

Pauline looked up and saw that David was winking at her and grinning a mischievous little grin.

"What's that?" she asked, but David just grinned. "C'mon, tell me. Oh, I know. Don't even tell me. I know. Uh-uh. No. You'll never get me to . . ."

"I haven't said a thing."

"I know. I know," Pauline said, nodding her head back and forth like a rebellious child. "You want me to write a book, right? Am I right? I'm right. Right?"

"Well, think about it. Actually I was thinking more in terms of your editing a collection of essays on kidney disease, maybe contributing one or two articles yourself. With a co-editor. And I'd be glad to help. It would be great experience for you. For Pete's sake, you know just about everything there is to know about kidney disease by now. You've been doing therapy at the renal center for almost four years now."

Pauline had been doing psychiatric consultations for renal dialysis patients for several years now. Many kidney patients have trouble adapting to the rigors of dialysis—the special dietary prescriptions, the hours and hours spent hooked up to a machine every week. Pauline's practical approach had helped many of them adjust to the dialysis treatment, while making her an expert. She knew their frustrations, their hopes, the burdens placed on their families by the chronic nature of the disease.

David was full of ideas. He pulled them out of his hat like a magician, handkerchief after handkerchief. What, sick? No, he didn't have the time. Every new project the two of them got started on added three more to his list. It reminded me of the television show, "Run for Your Life." Ben Gazzara is told he has six months to live; make the most of it. For David, making the most of it meant continuing his contributions to medical research.

It's funny about that television show. I remember so vividly what my father said when I explained what the show was all about. "See, this guy is real sick and his doctor told him he will live six months max, so he goes all around the world and does all this stuff," I explained. "No doctor can ever predict how long a patient will live. They shouldn't even try to," David said, unequivocally.

David and Pauline's heightened activity was certainly a way of running, but it was also a way of facing up to reality: David wanted to make damn sure Pauline secured that tenure. Not that he didn't trust her capabilities—he just wanted to give her an extra push to make doubly sure. With that security, he could go in peace.

The hard work paid off in December, when the NIH awarded David the $300,000 grant for his contraceptive research. It was a real boost for Dad and the entire family. The male contraceptive was a sexy topic and in the months to follow it became a hot item in the press. After the official statement was made, the news hit all the papers, science journals, and women's magazines. A unisex contraceptive! Which, in its final form, would be a nasal spray. "Sniff N'Sex," was the title of one article. "After all, an unwanted pregnancy is nothing to sneeze at!" wrote one journalist. The publicity was incredible, making it very easy to attract a group of male volunteers. Meanwhile, on the home front, we were inundated with articles relatives and friends had clipped out of South African and European journals. There were telephone calls from disk jockeys calling long-distance from all over the country. TV cameras showed up at the house; reporters kept the lines busy; even *Us* magazine came out to do a story and interviewed the whole family. Would men use it? Would women trust men to use it? "I'll have to leave that to the sociologists," David said. "Lots of work to do before then." He appeared on local television talk shows and on public radio. Everywhere he went he asked for volunteers to contact Vanderbilt Medical Center. He couldn't wait to get started on the project.

He was still swimming daily, but it was harder and harder for him to get in and out of the pool, in and out of his clothes, in and out of the shower, the dressing room, the car. Every morning the disability was there, waiting for him. No time off. No free weekends. The publicity was a release and a boost. He was a hero—a feminist scientist. He was featured in the *New York Times* and made the front page of the *Washington Post*. "He wants to put the birth control burden on men" was the title of one article. "Our Daddy is so famous!" Dana cried, but Leora was wary. She'd see something—a movement he made, or a gesture—and trail Mom out to the kitchen to question her.

David was running, but it was catching up with him. In January he bought a cane to help him get around. The new gadget seemed a cold intrusion on our warm home, but David played down its significance. He called it a "stick"—never a "cane"—and the euphemism glided by us. He was tiring more quickly now, and he began taking short, discreet afternoon naps either at his office or in the living room at home. He knew that soon he would have to be fitted for leg braces. The foot-drop had grown worse, and sometimes he almost tripped over his own feet. But he kept moving. He drove to Memphis to give a talk, flew to Pittsburgh to participate in a seminar, then hopped down to Mobile and over to Knoxville. Even in the anonymous eyes of the airport he was changing. We went to pick him up when he returned from Harvard, where he had delivered one of his outstanding lectures. It was about a young Israeli woman who not only lacked any trace of the female hormone FSH, but actually made antibodies to FSH! The miracle was that after years of therapy she had finally succeeded in getting pregnant. Dad loved telling the story . . .

The trail of passengers coming down the walkway thinned out to a trickle, but Dana and I were still waiting. No Daddy. Maybe he missed the plane, running Hairbreadth Harry time. "Everybody's off already," the steward assured us.

"Are you sure? Could you check?"

"Hey little lady, I know my business. Everyone's off the flight."

"Sure?"

"Yeah. Might be on the next one from Boston. Five-fifty, gate 12."

"No, he would have called."

"Well now, I tell you, everyone's off that flight except for one man walking with a limp, real slowly."

HEY.

"Hey, that's my father. That's who we were asking about."

"Oh," the steward said, giving us a funny look. "Oh. You should have said something."

A few days later a letter arrived for Dad from Dr. Crowley, the endocrinologist who had invited him to Harvard. "Just a brief note to congratulate you once again on your beautiful talk here. I have never gotten so many compliments about an invited guest speaker as I have about you . . . we are very eager to get you back for a little more prolonged stay next year." Dad's dynamic when he speaks: he stumbles up to the podium but when he gets there he is in control. He's center stage. Clear, elegant, vibrant. A star.

The invitations kept pouring in, but meanwhile, at the airport, even strangers knew something was fishy. David, and the rest of our family, by association, were slowly being pushed into the ranks of The Other. The Other was sick, different, and most of all, separate. People don't know how to talk to The Other, and they make strange assumptions. We noticed little things at first. A friendly hostess at the airport turned to Dana, asking "Would your friend like to use a wheelchair?" Why didn't she ask David himself? For fear he would be embarrassed? Or that perhaps his disability extended beyond the physical?

At the theater, something else happened. We would all be ushered in as a group, without even having our tickets checked or stubs pulled. Why? Disabled people are honest?

My parents rebelled against this regrouping and relabeling. They refused to be shunted off to the outer circle. They simply refused to go. They were still okay, still normal, still part of the crowd, even still among the movers and shakers. To prove it they gave dinner parties and made phone calls and chatted and kept up with people. They had parties and invited artists and newcomers and friends of friends they had just met. They were wonderful hosts, delightful and charming. Pauline served hors d'oeuvres and David even learned how to mix a few drinks. They showered their guests with news and tidbits of gossip and the-funniest-thing-happened-today stories. But their friends sensed a strangeness.

Something was going on. David and Pauline were trying too hard. The guests could sense it. A greediness, an avarice, a trying to get too much in too quickly. Even old friends felt uncomfortable. They felt something was expected of them, something they could not give. David and Pauline were gorging themselves. Pauline laughed a bit too loudly; David was a shade too witty. There was something off-balance, something off-key. And there was something very important that was not being said. It was deliberately left out of conversations, glossed over in introductions. Friends didn't know whether to ask David how he was doing or pretend they hadn't noticed anything was wrong. And yet it was so obvious something was wrong. But it was also obvious he didn't want to talk about it.

Then, at the end of an evening, after all the laughter and good cheer, the guests could see the strain on David's face as he clutched the arm-rests of his chair with his fists and hoisted himself up to mix someone a drink. Or he would say, "Help yourself." As the weeks went by, he no longer walked them to the door at the end of an evening. And he was always seated when they came in. A big smile on his face, a loud hello, but he wouldn't stand up. When he did stand up, he didn't stand up straight.

What did he take them for, fools? How long could he go on with this charade? And whom was he kidding, this proud man? Why couldn't he just be straight with them? It was more than back trouble, anyone could see that. You didn't have to be an expert.

Some people felt David was being dishonest with them. Why the pretense? Why was he trying to pull the wool over their eyes—didn't he trust them? Didn't he respect them enough to be frank with them? They needed to know what was going on. Why couldn't he just tell them?

My parents were losing touch. It wasn't that they were unaware, because they did pick up subtleties, nuances, innuendoes. But they were detached. They were so busy concentrating on keeping their lives going. It was like following an intricate dance pattern. Just one wrong step would get them out of synchronism with the music. They couldn't afford to make a mistake. They had to concentrate on the dance, on each and every step. They couldn't afford to spare any energy to look up and around them. They had to concentrate on the theme song—Normal Living.

Certainly their friends would understand. Surely it made sense. The ordinary rules of honesty and openness in friendship could be suspended for a while. This was just too painful to discuss. This was the easiest way for them to cope . . . the only way for them to cope. Some people need to talk and share all; some need to be quiet and let their friends take them away from their troubles on drifts of conversation. That was what David and Pauline needed. Surely their friends could understand.

PART **2**

Summertime

CHAPTER 1

Michael

By March Michael wanted to know what was going on. David had asked him to fly down for a weekend to drive him to Knoxville, where he could be fitted with ankle braces. He couldn't make the drive on his own. "Sure," Michael said, "I can work a Saturday and get a three-day weekend off. But what's this all about? C'mon, tell me. What's going on? Why don't you just tell me what's going on?" So David told him.

And Pauline said: Maybe that's what "ready" is, when they say, tell me. When it's gotten to the point of knowing, but not having the right name for it. If there is such a thing as ready.

Elisabeth Kübler-Ross was the first to describe the five stages of grief: denial, anger, bargaining, depression, acceptance. Usually they occur within a whirlwind of emotion, obscured by the constant and overwhelming sense of loss and grief. In Michael the stages were distinct and easily identifiable, primarily because of his particular circumstances.

First, denial. Michael didn't understand. Oh, he understood all right—on one level. If you asked him what was wrong, he could say, "My father has ALS. It's a progressive degenerative nerve disease." He could probably explain the physiology of the illness and mutter something about statistical prognostic chances. But it was all academic. The knowledge was controlled, detached, intellectualized. He was operating only on that one level, the first paper-thin layer outermost in the mind. Then there was a block.

His father, sick? Okay, so he's got a limp. Big deal. He's not sick—
not deathly sick anyway. Look at him: laughing, writing away at
his desk. An invalid? Paralyzed? What, Dad? Nah. Can't even
picture it. It's crazy. You just don't understand: Dad always puts
things to right, fixes, heals, cures, glues it back together again. A
doctor, for Pete's sake. He makes things better. He'll find a way
out of this mess. He's so smart; he'll figure it out.

Denial is a survival instinct. You never really get past it.
"Dad just walks slowly because he isn't in a hurry," I used to say
to myself. "He's so smart—he's just trying to prove a point." Or
"He isn't losing weight—he's always been slim and trim." Denial
doesn't entirely deserve the bad reputation it has acquired. Both
positive and negative forms of denial exist. Positive denial protects
you; gives you a chance to get used to the news gradually. It
breaks the fall. Later, when you're used to the knowledge, it's a
forgetfulness, a pretense, a rest. You couldn't live without it, not
any semblance of a normal life. You'd freak out. Wouldn't be
able to go to school, go to work, make dinner, carry on a life.
Like blinders on a horse, you need it to keep going forward.

After denial there is the anger that comes with recognition.
Anger is easy, and there is so much anger—at the disease, at
chance, fate, bad luck, this life. But there's no one to blame.
The patient is the nearest available target. He's "handling it the
wrong way." He has a "cancer personality." He is being "punished
by God." We have to explain it somehow, because we run our
lives on cause and effect, and an aberration makes us uneasy.
The patient becomes the scapegoat of our ignorance, and we
achieve two things at once: a cathartic release for our grief and
sometimes even a temporary respite from our painful love for the
source of the sorrow.

"It is necessary to become a bit angry with patients who are
dying, if only as a way of separating from someone in whom
one has invested a good bit of time and probably a good bit of
caring," Alice Trillin, a cancer patient, wrote in the the *New
England Journal of Medicine*. "We all do this to people who are
sick. I remember being terribly angry with my mother. Somehow
I needed to think that it was her fault that she was sick, because
her illness frightened me so much. I was also angry with my
friend who died of cancer. I felt that she had let me down, that

perhaps she hadn't fought hard enough. It was important for me to find reasons for her death, to find things she might have done to cause it, as a way of separating myself from her and as a way of thinking that I would somehow have behaved differently, that I would somehow have been able to stay alive."

People who care try to understand the anger; people who don't use it as an excuse and a short cut. All the books say "it's natural" but it stills feels terrible when you love someone. Michael was stuck up in Chicago, five hundred miles away; Mom, Dad, and the little girls were holding the fort, and time was running out. Damn it. Dad had known in June. Two months—a good two months—before he started the job in Chicago. Why didn't he let Michael know back then? What was he supposed to do now—quit his job? No, Dad wouldn't hear of it. Damn, Dad always had to do everything his way.

David used to argue with him. "You've got a job to do and that's all that matters," he said over and over again. "Do your job and do it well and learn as much as you can. I refuse to let this illness get in the way of your career. My motto has been for us to live our lives as close to the normal way as possible. You've got your own life. I'm sick but your life goes on—if all goes well it'll be a long and healthy life. If you come home and start hanging around here I'll have to die just so you can get back to your life. Don't you see? I'm not going to sit and watch you be a bum. If you come down for the weekend as often as you can, and keep in touch, that's enough. This isn't acute illness. You're a real help when you're around."

So Michael proceeded to Bargaining. He was still in Chicago but he got home often for a long weekend. A typical weekend: Friday afternoon he mows the lawn, makes fettucini for supper. Saturday morning does the grocery shopping, buys Dana and Leora a record ("Just felt like it, that's all"), plants a garden in the afternoon. Toward evening he starts cleaning out the basement. Early up on Sunday to finish, take Dana and Leora to a matinee before his flight out. Michael loves projects: fixing doors, changing window screens, scrubbing the fridge. As if he's pleading: "If I do all this? And clean out the garage? And throw a pancake brunch into the bargain? Then will Dad get better?" When I drove out to Chicago from Oberlin to visit him he spoiled me: a Second City show, drinks on him, chocolate fondue at a snazzy French restaurant. Hoarding amusements like armaments, before battle.

Then, Depression. Inertia, listlessness, loss of direction, feelings of meaninglessness. Loss of appetite or "gorging"; drowsiness or insomnia; sometimes loss of libido, impotence. Boredom, alienation, isolation, loneliness. Michael's girlfriend, Ellen, had gone out to school in California and he felt stranded. No one to talk to; no one to listen; no shock absorbers. He tried to fill the gap with lots of letters and expensive phone calls. After work he jogged around the lake, hitting the still icy wind. Then back to the apartment to drop on the couch. No energy. Habits kept him in line: a couple of loads of laundry, cook up a batch of soup, change the linen. Sometimes he called the folks, just to hear their voices. He sounded bad but he'd never admit it, saying he had just called to see how they were managing. "You don't sound good, Michael. Are you okay?" "Yeah, just a bad connection. Sounds far off or something."

An idea started forming in his mind. Sunny California. He could join Ellen at Stanford, at the business school out there. They had an excellent health management program—the number one MBA place in the country.

But this time David said "No." Stanford was just too far away. Yes, Harvard's far but Michael could catch a plane and be home in a matter of hours. Piedmont even had a Hopscotch Special, $169.

Trivial difference, Michael said.

That two hours can make the difference between getting home for the weekend or not though, David said, and besides— Harvard is Harvard.

But, Michael said, Harvard is number two in the top ten; Stanford is number one. In last year's ratings of business schools. . . .

I don't want you that far away, David said.

But if you had told me in June I could've been in Nashville this whole past year and next year, Michael argued.

You looked for a job here, didn't you? You didn't find anything you wanted.

The debate ended with David retreating on his position. He thought it over and decided that Michael was right, that his ban on Stanford Business School was inconsistent with his "as normal

as possible" philosophy, and he told Michael to send off the
application "with my blessing." That was unusual in itself because
David could be pretty determined at times, and on this issue in
particular the rest of us tended to agree with him. But David
realized that Michael's relationship with Ellen was at stake—a
coast-to-coast relationship seemed implausible, if not impossible—
and that played a potentially large role in Michael's future. Then
a funny thing happened, and the decision was taken out of their
hands. Michael wasn't accepted to Stanford! He'd be going to
Harvard after all. He was disappointed, as was Dad. In retrospect
I think things turned out for the best and Michael was glad he
could get home in three hours. In a strange way his Stanford
idea was a final last clutch at denial. If he was out on the West
Coast, things couldn't be all that bad.

The last stage is Acceptance. Still, acceptance is ephemeral; it
comes in momentary flashes. When you try to hold on to it it
eludes you, disappears like a spark. Fact: David is going to die.
After that, there is hope. Exercise, lecithin, experimental drugs
from across the Iron Curtain, scientific miracles, last-minute
breakthroughs. Up in Chicago, Michael took lecithin tablets
daily, as though to spur David on. Maybe it would improve his
memory. It had sharpened David's—he could recall the plays he
and Pauline saw while they were dating, who acted what parts,
snippets of dialogue, the funny thing that happened afterward
when they went out for coffee. She draws a blank. It's incredible.
And you think, he's so smart, he'll figure something out.

CHAPTER 2

Roni

On May 17, 1980, I handed in my last exam of the semester. I was home free. I was all packed; the last thing to come down from my wall was the blown-up photo from *Us* magazine showing Dad holding a test tube up to the light. I would be flying to Nashville in a couple of hours. But something was bugging me. I didn't know what it was, couldn't pin it down. Something a friend had said. His mother had a slipped disk too, and we always compared notes. But something was wrong. His mother had pain. Terrible pain, he said. Dad swore that he didn't. Well that was easy to explain away: Dad was protecting us. But Bill's mother was planning to undergo surgery. It was the best thing—all of the doctors agreed. Risky, but preferable to . . . well, a wheelchair. I cross-examined him. What were the chances of success? Why didn't my father have surgery? Well, why did he think he didn't? Was his mother swimming? Well what, was my father a nut? I knew his condition was deteriorating. They never said anything but I could tell by Mom's tone of voice on the phone. Faint. Evasive. Like an overseas call ten years ago. He was getting worse, and they didn't want to tell me. But I could picture the disk, bone bearing down on the fragile wisp of a nerve. Any moment, snap.

The next day, back home in Nashville, Mom told me the truth. We went to the supermarket, and on the way home she turned into a side street.

"Hey, where are you going?" I asked her.

"Oh, there's a house here for sale, I just wanted to take a look. . . ." she said, in that evasive tone. And then she pulled the car over and parked on the shoulder of the road. "I need to talk to you alone and quietly." After a long pause she said slowly and sadly, "Dad's condition is progressive."

"What does that mean?"

"It's a progressive thing. It keeps getting worse."

"Well, I can tell that much," I said cavalierly, not wanting to understand.

"Not just in the legs. All over. It's a progressive degenerative neurological disease. It's terminal," Mom said in a hard voice. I crumpled. She waited a few minutes, I don't know how long, but it didn't seem long enough. Then she started the engine. "Come on. Wipe your face—there's tissues under the seat. I don't want anyone to see you've been crying. Look how brave he is. You have to be brave too. I know it's hard . . . but we're just going to try to live as normally as possible for as long as we can."

I cried a lot, that summer. I'd say that on the average, I cried twice a week for the next year and a half. But you get the crying out and go on with it. I survived that summer. I kept busy. I took three English courses, waited tables part-time, and did volunteer work. I listened to everything Dad said, memorizing every word, every moment. It was as if he had always known: "Life is too short to fight; life is too short to be sad." So I wasn't sad. If Dad could do it, then hell, so could I. I owed it to him. I owed it to Dana and Leora too. They still didn't know, at least not consciously. They were around it all the time, they saw Dad stumbling, they sensed something was amiss. But for them it was still normal living; we were creating normal living for them a little while longer. So we managed to laugh. Dad brought the family to eat at the restaurant one evening, and I waited on them. He left me a ten-dollar tip on a thirty-dollar bill, and on the way out he said to the manager, "I don't know who that waitress is but she's excellent, efficient, and very courteous. Hang on to her. Hell, give her a raise."

That summer he was walking with the cane in one hand, a rail or chair or wall in the other. He planned his route by the landmarks he could grasp. It was denial—negative denial. And it was getting dangerous. He was still driving, that foot slow as lead on the accelerator. Stop signs, red lights: he had to plan ahead. He tried not to stray from familiar routes. We could have insisted, or refused, or demanded—but we all participated in the denial, and the control was so important to him. Being able to drive meant he was independent, and he wanted to maintain his independence. He wouldn't even consider a wheelchair. "But what if there's a fire and we have to get you out in a hurry?" So Mom bought one, a fold-up model that sat in the pantry behind the door where no one could see it. If the wheel slipped out when you were there getting potatoes for dinner you had a fright. The chair was the beginning of the end, we all knew that. *There is no regeneration of the already damaged nerves.* By not exercising you merely compound the wasting of muscle that's already taking place. Sit down and you leave the legs to rot. So David kept walking. Walking, often falling, and picking himself up again.

Falling is a big part of the illness, albeit a strangely silent part. It's never mentioned by experts, in textbooks. It's a quiet part only the patients and the family experience. Only the patient and the family know the cracked ribs, those red blotches on the chest, the heating pad for the pain, six or eight weeks until it heals. And the worry at every step. Watching, ready to run. Each step of the foot monitored, observed, measured. "I have fallen down in every room in my house: in the bathroom, the bedroom, the kitchen, the dining room, the lavatory, down the stairs and up the stairs," one ALS patient wrote. "In April I fell at home and had to go into the emergency ward for four or five stitches," wrote another. "About a week later I fell again, in my office, which has a hard linoleum-covered floor, and broke three or four bones in my face and my right hand. I was hospitalized then for another week."

Obviously this man should not have been walking. But it's easier for an outsider to say. Some people need an authoritative voice to break through their own denial. I know we did. "No. You cannot walk any longer." Or, "No. It isn't safe. You cannot do it." But Fitzgerald was nowhere in sight. He had passed David in the street and he didn't even point out that David was using the cane incorrectly. Maybe he didn't notice; maybe he didn't even know. The stick was too long, and David was holding it in the wrong hand. If it were shortened a bit he could get more leverage, and if he held it in the right hand, the hand of the stronger leg, that would create a tripodlike effect. Later when he went to Knoxville with Michael, the physical therapist had explained this to him.

As for me, I started reading. One day a newspaper article caught my eye. It was a guy in Miami, a cure for multiple sclerosis, a potion made from snake venom. Dad wasn't impressed. But that didn't stop me. I went on reading, gobbling up Norman Cousins' *Anatomy of an Illness* and *Getting Well Again* by Carl and Stephanie Simonton. These books echoed an attitude toward illness that I had seen actively expressed by my father every day, i.e., that when every iota of your energy and will be devoted to living and creating, illness simply cannot triumph. It seemed a natural idea, almost common sense. "But of course."

These ideas were not new to me. Up at Oberlin I had girlfriends who practiced natural birth control. They blocked out all artificial lights at night so their bodies would ebb and flow with the moon's rhythm. With mortar and pestle they crushed herbs which they slipped into capsules and ate with their granola at breakfast. Black cohash to induce menstruation; jasmine and chamomile for cramps. Self-prescribed placebos, I thought to myself now. I had always been skeptical but they were patient with me—after all, both my parents were medical doctors. They convinced me I had been duped by the modern gods of objectivity and scientific method. Not everything can be measured and observed, they told me. Historically, the mind-body split is a recent invention—a technological ploy, an AMA plot. The medical community had robbed us of our mental powers simply by teaching us they did not exist. Awareness of power is power.

I checked myself: was this an oversimplification? But no: placeboes were concrete evidence of the positive powers of belief. And when you laugh, endorphins—a form of morphine which humans make naturally—are released from the brain. To Norman Cousins' vitamin C and Marx Brothers films, David had his daily lecithin milkshakes and "M*A*S*H" shows. Of course, we found out later that lecithin did not work the way my parents had hoped it would. First David reached his own private conclusion.

After taking it for a whole year he decided that placebo or not, it was not producing any beneficial effects. The stuff was so hard to get down that he really couldn't justify taking it any longer. It was grainy and heavy and he often felt nauseous after his daily dose. It just wasn't worth it. Later on the research confirmed his instinctive conclusion when he and Pauline found no evidence of elevated acetylcholine levels in the subjects who had eaten the horrible stuff (the results were published in the *Journal of Clinical Psychiatry*). But it shouldn't have mattered. David was active, creative, and productive. He was swimming and biking. And he didn't devote himself to his illness—he led a balanced lifestyle. And he had so much fight left in him—how could he possibly lose?

We were going to lick this thing. I was convinced.

CHAPTER 3

Anger

That was my first phase—denial. Dad will get better, no problem. But what if he didn't? I needed a back-up. If he didn't, it meant—according to my theory—that he didn't want to hard enough. And I just couldn't buy that. I couldn't lay any blame at his feet. Over the three months I was home that summer I watched closely for signs of deterioration. It seemed he was throwing out his leg more to take the same size step. Or was he? It was hard to tell, hard to measure. If he was getting worse, what did it mean? Somehow I had to tie it in neatly with my holistic healing theories, while at the same time making excuses for possible failure. My books told me that a "recent crisis" or "stressful period," left unresolved, could spark off an illness. If I could pinpoint a crisis, that would at least take some of the responsibility off David's shoulders. I needed a scapegoat. Some-one—or something—to blame. I needed a focus for my frustra-tion. Damn it, I was angry. This thing had intruded on our lives for no reason; it hovered over us, coming down on us slowly and insidiously, threatening to descend with full force at any moment. If we could fight it off, fine; if we couldn't, I needed more informa-tion in order to create a sense of order. The illness was horrible; not knowing where it came from or why, made it utterly in-tolerable. It unleashed senselessness and chaos on everything. I needed an answer to "why." So I created one. I found a recent "crisis" to take the blame.

* * *

In 1968 our family had immigrated to Israel from Baltimore. My parents had every intention of making it a permanent move and building a new home there, but from the first day there were problems. They had always harbored Zionist dreams. The ideology of the early settlers appealed to them, with its special blend of socialism and equality, independence and freedom of a people in their own land. When Israel emerged strong and triumphant in 1967 (after the Six-Day War), Pauline and David decided it was now or never.

Unfortunately, the realities didn't match the dreams. At least not entirely. So in June, 1968, our family's tempestuous love-hate relationship with Israel began. When we arrived we set about learning the language, the exotic Middle-East smells and spices, the back alleys and shortcuts of Jerusalem, our new home. We enjoyed peaceful afternoons on the kibbutz with our cousins, and heated arguments about politics over coffee and homemade cake. Every weekend there was something new to explore: an archaeology dig where Crusader ruins had just been unearthed, a nature hike through a desert oasis, a walk through the old walled city of Jerusalem. But the '67 war had unleashed some ugly elements in Israel: a strident militarism and much internal disagreement over the future of the West Bank and its inhabitants, the Palestinians. There were fewer than three million Jews in Israel, but they fought among themselves on almost every topic. The Ashkenazim didn't like the Sephardim, who didn't like the kibbutzniks, who didn't agree with the moshavniks, all of whom resented the extremist Orthodox Jews, who threw stones at the Jewish cars passing by their neighborhood on the Sabbath.

"Two Jews, three opinions," is the saying. It made life exciting but produced a lot of tension, and the tension extended to my parents' workplace, the Hadassah Medical Center. Competition between the professionals was fierce at Hadassah, and emotions ran high. But it was more than just a clash of temperaments with my parents' genteel Anglo-Saxon heritage. Even before David arrived, one of the Israeli doctors had warned him, "It's a mine field." And it was. The doctors resented one another's successes and jealously guarded their hospital "turf," their special privileges and duties. David was doing extremely well with his research.

He was publishing in international journals and speaking at all the European conferences. Patients had heard about his gentle manner and expertise, and they left the doctors they had frequented for years. The course David taught at the medical school was standing-room-only. The other doctors couldn't take it. They refused to cooperate with him on research projects. Some stopped greeting him in the halls. The faculty parties were so tense David and Pauline avoided them altogether. And David had little support from the hospital administration. It was a slap in the face for David, who had gone to live with other Jews to build a Jewish state.

We left Israel in 1973. It was now 1980, several years later, and I hated those doctors. With a vengeance. I despised them, and I brooded on my hatred. I held them personally responsible for my father's sickness. Years earlier I might have said their behavior was "human nature," and maybe Dad had been a bit arrogant, and not totally blameless himself. But now I accepted no excuses whatsoever. The Hadassah doctors, many of whom I knew, or whose children I had gone to school with, became monstrous caricatures of human beings in my eyes. It became a total obsession with me. I fantasized about meeting one of them, and saying just the right words to rip him to shreds. In my mind I relived my father's days at Hadassah, feeling the pain and isolation he must have felt. I rehearsed scenarios over and over again in my mind, and I chided myself for not being sensitive and helpful to David back then, I dwelled on it, talked about it and cursed. Whenever the subject of the Middle East came up in conversation it set me off on a tirade, unleashing a barrage of accusations and recriminations. It wasn't just Hadassah—the hospital was merely a microcosm. The whole country was vicious, mean, a cesspool of rot and corruption.

It was an irrational response, excessive and overblown. I knew that even then. I saw the looks of bewilderment on my friends' faces—the "there she goes again" looks—but I couldn't stop myself. And somehow, the outbursts must have had a soothing, cathartic effect on me. I always felt much better after one of my verbal attacks.

My private little war on Israel was not limited to a war of words. Far from it. I was going to personally embargo the country.

Israel encourages and needs new immigrants, and ever since my family left in 1973 I had intended to return. Now I resolved I would never go back. I couldn't, even if I wanted to. How could I return to a country I held responsible for David's horrible illness? Crazy, yes. But it didn't seem so at the time. At the time it gave me a great feeling of power. I was not impotent in the face of this illness. I could still avenge my father's pain. It didn't matter that no one knew or cared whether I lived in Israel or in the United States I knew. It was a personal, private vendetta. I was holding out. And the funniest thing about this crazy, irrational mode of thought is that it kept me sane for a long time. Anger can be very healthy: it keeps you focused so you always know what side you're on. I carried these feelings—alternately complacent and assured of David's recovery, and angry and resentful toward Israel—around with me for more than a year.

Most of the time it was easiest just to fool myself David was getting better, not worse. Everyone goes through crises in their lifetime. What counts is how the crises are resolved. My books told me that. They said it was important not to "bottle up" your feelings. I recalled marathon discussions during our first year back in the States, during which we all expressed our feelings about leaving Israel. Anyway, that was a long time ago, I told myself. Six years between Israel and the first symptoms. More to the point, Dad himself wasn't bitter about the Israel experience. "Sure, if you want to be bitter you can blame just about anything. You can blame Israel, but you have to remember, it wasn't a wholly negative experience. There are some beautiful things there. It just wasn't for us."

And in a sense, I told myself, it wasn't even a question of what precipitated the illness. It was a question of fighting back. And Dad was just too alive to be dying.

No. I was convinced. We're going to lick this thing.

CHAPTER 4

At the Beach

"Sometimes I wonder," my mother said one day, "I wonder if I appreciated him enough when he was well. Those picky little things. We didn't call him Hairbreadth Harry for nothing. He was late all the time. He'd show up for a six o'clock movie at six, even when we were dating. But he's so wonderful. Can you imagine anyone else with this awful illness? If I had it, I'd be impossible. I'd drive you all mad. He accepts help so graciously. And he used to be so independent. It's easier for a woman, to be helped, to have things done for her. Sometimes I wish it were me. I don't know how I'll go on without him. It's been the two of us for so long. It was never a question. All the divorce nowadays . . . we did everything together. We enjoyed each other. I never wanted to be alone."

It's the truth, not the product of retroactive sentimentality. They've always been together, a tight fit, yin and yang. When she pleads, he's calm; when she blusters, he grins. They balance each other out. Both sharp, like ginger and garlic, but distinct: straight-sharp, with a twang. He has blue eyes; she, high cheekbones. They go together. Both love classical music, good writing, a sense of humor about life. Even now, she complained to him about the new hospital, how there are never any elevators, you have to wait for fifteen minutes—what if there's an emergency? See what aggravation my illness has spared me? he asked.

When my mother and I talked, I would assure her she would

never be alone. Never. You've got a career, and a good position, I would tell her. You've always had your own life. Besides, I would tell her, there are four of us; you can come live with each one for three months out of every year if you want. And I would laugh. "That way we won't even get tired of you. Anyway, you're a lot stronger than you think you are. Know that?" And I would think: she held it in all that time. A whole year. She didn't come crying to us. She could have. There was one incident in particular I remembered. It was before I had known the diagnosis. We were at the pool. "It's so sad," Mom had said, watching Dad struggle. I still thought he had a slipped disk. "God damn, Mom," I'd said, "you're really exaggerating. He has a back problem. So what? He could have—cancer or something." She hadn't said a word. Just looked at me.

We went to a modern dance performance. One of the dances was done to the tune of "He's not heavy, he's my brother." Mom nudged me with her elbow. "You can think of it as 'He's not heavy, he's my David,' " she whispered. I knew she was worrying herself sick, having difficulty getting to sleep at nights; yesterday her heart skipped a beat. "Arrhythmia," she said, knowing that widows have a higher mortality rate than the population at large. "Even when something good happens, I'll be feeling good about it and then I'll remember," she said. "I'll pick a fight with him, over nothing, I realize later. Just half thinking that if he gets irritated enough he'll get up and stomp out of the room." But he never did, so she immersed herself in her work, planning seminars, revising papers for publication; anything to ward off decay. She had decided to go ahead with a book on kidney failure with a colleague, and the two used to sit with David for hours over manuscripts: editing, condensing, reconstructing, rearranging.

Mom held us together. She planted a garden: tomatoes, eggplants, cucumbers, rosemary. She had the downstairs renovated; moved the master bedroom to the first floor so Dad could get to it more easily. He had to rest in the afternoons now; it was crazy for him to use up all his energy just getting to and from the bedroom. A Jacuzzi was put in the bathroom—the warm sprays eased the spasm and the stiffness. Pauline picked out a bright green and yellow flowered wallpaper for the bathroom. Things weren't going to get run down because Daddy's sick. We weren't going to fall apart. We weren't going to lower our standards.

We went to the beach at Hilton Head in South Carolina for vacation. The sand there is smooth and packed, but Dad stayed by the pool. Every morning someone would be nominated to get out early and reserve an umbrella; underneath it on the table we stacked *Time* and *New Republic* magazines, towels, suntan lotion, a jug of ice tea, and a hard-backed chair for Dad. We borrowed each other's copies of *The World According to Garp* and *Anatomy of an Illness*. Every morning Mike lowered Dad into the pool. He swam twice every day. "It's not the length of life that's important, it's the quality. Quality, not quantity," Dad said, as we were sitting out by the pool one day. "I've had a good life." And I watched as he brushed a fly away from his chin. His fingers swept across his face. They appeared frail, uncoordinated, but I thought it must be my imagination.

Uncle Jack came to spend a week with us. It was the first time he'd ever been to America. "Don't underestimate Jack's grief," Dad warned us. "They say losing a child is hardest, then a spouse comes in close second, then a parent. I've always been like a son to Jack. He provided a roof over my head all through medical school, and he paid for whatever the bursaries left out. He was always proud of me, never jealous. As if I were his son. And he never had children of his own. I'm sure it never occurred to him that he might outlive me. We talked about that; I think that's important. I explained the realities of the illness to him. And he sees we're not living out the days in ashes and sackcloth." When we took Jack back to the airport he leaned on me. "Be brave," he whispered as we watched Dad fling his legs in front of him, like stilts attached at the hip. The legs flounced and flopped onto the floor. And Jack looked at me and asked, "Why'd it have to be him?"

It was the summer of *10* and I did my hair up in Bo Derek braids. Leora ran off with some friends she'd found on the beach. Dana bought a new bathing suit and burned where the tan lines changed. She and Mom took long walks on the beach at low tide, walks Mom used to take with Dad. In the evening Mike and I would cook up vegetarian dishes: eggplant almond enchiladas and mushroom curry. After dinner we played word games. Our favorite: Dictionary. You find a word that no one knows, and everyone has to come up with a definition. Then you read them all aloud and vote on which you think is the real one.

It was summer in slow motion. We were living on hot air and Norm Cousins.

"I think I'm stabilizing," Dad said one day, as we were sitting under the umbrella. "I think the swimming's done a helluva lot of good for me. And the lecithin. . . ."

"Stable" was a key vocabulary word in our household that summer. Dad is "stable." His condition is "stabilizing." He's not getting better but he's "stable."

"That lecithin is awful stuff but the swimming, swimming is a real pleasure," Dad told us. "When you're inactive and your mobility is restricted, to be in a medium where you're virtually weightless and have agility is a real pleasure. Aside from the physical therapy it's a psychological respite. My body isn't a burden in the water. . . ."

But sometimes he barely lifted that left arm out of the water. Other times it fell just as it was about to break the surface, as if he'd dropped it.

My mind drifted off and I remembered what I had dreamt the night before. I dreamt Dad was well. He took us out to eat at my restaurant. After a hearty meal, lots of protein, he got up without the stick. It had fallen behind the table and he bent over to pick it up, twirled it in the air and did a tap dance. He didn't need to lean on it, he just used it to feel the texture of the floor ahead of him to know what kind of step to take.

"I'm telling you all this because I think if I keep this up I'll be in good shape. If I can just keep on going like this . . ."

The two-year point was crucial. At least that was what Dad kept telling us: that the disease does most of its damage during the first two years, then it eases off. Most experts refuse to predict, because the disease varies so much from person to person. But Dad was convinced that if he could just make it through the first two years, he would have made it through the worst. I counted the months. It was August. Nine more months to go, and then he might have a good five or ten years. Nine more months with my fingers crossed.

"I don't have any secrets," Dad said. "Hell, we've made a lot of mistakes. But everything we've learned we've figured out by trial and error. The doctors have been of no help, with the exception of Brewster. Fitzgerald isn't supportive. He's been incommunicado. He never calls, he just wrote me off, right from the start. It's not that he's malicious, but doctors aren't trained to deal with patients whom they cannot cure. It's a very real and very worrying gap in the training of physicians. They're divorced from the practical day-to-day considerations of living with a debilitating illness while still maintaining a modicum of dignity. And in this illness that's what counts. Because there is no cure.

"They put a dreadful connotation on ALS, in brochures given out by commendable institutions. They say there's no possibility of recovering lost movements. They say, 'ALS is a progressive disease and in the next few months and years the following things will happen to you.' Maybe they will, but I know from my own experience I've seen improvement. If you've lost the muscle it's not gone forever. I don't know how long the improvement will last, but it's an objective mark of improvement, and if it happened to me it can happen to others. People shouldn't have the notion that the muscle is lost forever—it will determine all subsequent activities, they'll give up on it. There's no magic—you have to exercise diligence, and be patient.

"And you have to remember the rules of the game. You're fighting a dragon. He's got the upper hand but you are not defenseless. With the combination of physical and psychological support methods you can make the illness livable, productive, and happy. It may sound strange but you can be happy even within the sadness of the disease. The sadness is underlying and it always prevails. But happiness has not disappeared from our lives. We're in a war; we fight the war as best we can. It's a communal effort that hopefully will be beneficial for all. We don't brood on the past; we get on with the present. There's no point in being Pollyanna-ish—it's a tough, brutal disease. But there's no point in giving in. It's much easier to give up, to say 'it's incurable' and wait passively for the inevitable. But that's negativistic. It leads to decay, to secondary complications: urinary infections, pneumonia, and ultimately death. You've got to fight and fight intelligently. Fight within the rules of the war. The rules are that you're fighting a defensive battle. But that shouldn't mean not to put up a defense. Diet, exercise, and rest are beneficial: and you can see their effects."

CHAPTER 5

A Day for David

That summer, it seemed, we had held death at bay. The threat had not dissipated, but we had held it at arm's length, had contained it, put it on ice. At the end of the summer lay our reward—the two-day David Rabin lectureship, a tribute to David from his colleagues and friends at Vanderbilt.

The David Rabin lectureship was the brainchild of Dr. Grant Liddle, Chief of Medicine at Vanderbilt and one of the driving forces behind David's recruitment to the university. Dr. Liddle was one of the first to whom David had confided his illness. Dad felt he owed it to him. That was the key to the special relationship between the two men—"mutual respect," Dad called it. Most of the doctors at Vanderbilt feared and revered Liddle, a brilliant scientist who ran the school with an iron hand and who, legend had it, had never been seen smiling in public. Not so David. The other doctors were always asking David to pass on messages and requests to Liddle for them—"C'mon, he'll listen to you." And it was true, Liddle did have a soft spot for David. When he learned of the illness, he was beside himself. Didn't know what to do, and couldn't do enough. He started dropping by the house in the evening, bringing tapes and records of his favorite operas. He offered to take rounds for David six months of the year, so as to ease his responsibilities at work. But he needed to do something bigger than that, something indelible. At first he planned the lectureship as a one-time affair, but some friends gathered enough funds to make it an annual symposium with a permanent place on the Vanderbilt calendar.

We all knew the lectureship was a big deal. We'd heard of "memorial lectures" but this was different and an even greater honor. The idea was for David to invite a lecturer of his choice and devote two whole days to talks and seminars on a chosen topic. David invited as the guest speaker his old friend and a wonderful lecturer from the National Institutes of Health, Jesse Roth. Several of our friends arranged social affairs around the academic events on Thursday and Friday—a party on Wednesday, a cocktail party Thursday, a formal sit-down dinner with Cornish hens, salmon-colored napkins, and matching roses on Friday. Not to mention the pastry breakfasts and buffet lunches hosted by the endocrine division.

On Wednesday morning Dr. Liddle opened the symposium with an eloquent introduction: "When Dr. Rabin joined our faculty as director of the division of endocrinology five years ago, we knew we were recruiting a star in world endocrinology on the basis of his published work and on the basis of his absolutely spectacular performance as a lecturer at various national and international forums. We did not know, however, the full measure of our good fortune. During the past six years we've been impressed with the genius of the technical expertise and the conceptual contributions that he has made to our diabetes research program. We've been impressed by the world-renowned innovations he has brought to clinical physiology in the area of reproductive physiology; we've been impressed by the great sophistication he's added to clinical research programs in pituitary physiology. Indeed, the breadth of his understanding of endocrinology makes it understandable that he's been capable, with the collaboration of a former Vanderbilt associate, Dr. McKenna, to produce a textbook of endocrinology authored by themselves alone.

"His excellence as a teacher of course is legendary to this audience. He has attracted more clinical fellows into endocrinology than we have ever had before and it is no exaggeration to say that under his guidance endocrinology at Vanderbilt has reached a level that has been unprecedented, and I believe it is safe to say that the endocrinology program here now is unsurpassed by any in the world.

"But that is not an adequate description of this remarkable man. Everyone with whom he comes in contact comes to admire and love David Rabin. He is a marvelous preceptor of young academics, and he is an invaluable collaborator of established investigators. But although he is very intense in cultivating the interests of his colleagues; and although he is totally devoted to his family; although he does everything possible for the advancement of scientific endocrinology; and although he is unstinting in his compassionate care for his patients; although he is completely loyal to this university and has won innumerable dear and distinguished friends in the community; and although he has steadily grown in professional prestige through election to all of the important professional societies in this country; David Rabin is a man who is personally completely unselfish. . . . He has made a lasting imprint on all, and the many who have known him, many who have only known him through his published works. He is a man with tremendous courage, one who truly loves life and all that is good in this world. He stands tall among us as an ideal role model, as a teacher, a physician, a scientist, a man, and a friend. And it is quite appropriate that we have established a David Rabin lectureship in endocrinology."

When Liddle finished speaking the president of the medical school senior class got up and presented David with a Vanderbilt chair. "David Rabin is without a doubt one of the most outstanding lecturers the students at Vanderbilt have had the privilege of engaging with," he said. "His presentations are noted for their clarity, and impart a true sense of understanding and energy. He has been a good friend of the students at all levels of relationships, as a teacher, advisor, and friend. It is these things which make David Rabin special to us, and it is with great honor and humility that we present him with this Vanderbilt chair. On the back there is a plaque which reads, 'David Rabin, MD, an excellent teacher and warm friend of the Vanderbilt Medical School, September 3, 1980.' We are proud, and we are inspired."

But a somber undertone accompanied the merriment. "I have mixed feelings about all these parties," Mom said. "It's really not a happy occasion." She wasn't referring only to the illness. There was something else as well. Between the various parties and dinners, she and David had managed to invite just about everyone they knew in Nashville. Again we felt the sense of unease and discomfort we were just beginning to identify among our friends and acquaintances. There were a few people in particular, who came to the parties, drank and ate, but never said a word to David all night. David, trapped in his chair, was impotent to approach them. Several times at the parties Dana, Leora, Mike, or I would glance over to see him—the guest of honor—sitting all alone in his chair. Quickly we would dispatch a guard to sit by his side, on the pretense of bringing him a plate full of cheese and a glass of juice.

On the second day of the lecture Dr. Roth presented David with a book of color reprints of a thousand masterpieces from the National Gallery of Art in Washington. "For an appreciator of excellence, and a creator of excellence," he said, explaining his choice of a gift. And I realized that David had been at the peak of his career when the illness hit him. It made me think of the JFK memorial on the outskirts of Jerusalem. The memorial is a building shaped like the bottom trunk of a thick healthy oak, axed down in its prime by a ruthless killer. David, as usual, had planned ahead and brought dark glasses to hide his tears.

CHAPTER 6

Pariah

We woke up from that blissful summer with a start.

We could no longer ignore it. Strange things were happening. Little things, subtle things, things you couldn't always put your finger on. Human relationships cannot be quantified; the warmth in a person's voice cannot be measured. But estrangement can be felt, sensed with a sixth sense. Even phone calls cannot be counted, but after a while one grows wary when too many people are too busy to visit or not at home, and the phone does not ring as often as it once did. When the six weeks between evenings with friends stretch to six months. When conversation is kept light-hearted and small talk dares go no further. At first we thought we were being paranoid. And we didn't talk about it, even among ourselves. How could we? There were no words for it in our vocabulary. Whatever it was, we had known about it before. We had probably done it ourselves. In a sense, we took it for granted. It was an integral part of our culture, an unwritten code agreed upon by all but the victims.

Perhaps we had expected it ever since David became ill.

People were avoiding us.

It was happening everywhere: in the corridors of the hospital, in Dana and Leora's classrooms, at movie theaters before the lights went out. In the supermarket, at the bakery, in line at the bookstore. People slinking around corners, looking straight ahead to avoid eye contact, pretending to be self-absorbed. It happened after dinner, before Grand Rounds, throughout cocktail parties. In restaurants, at the park, in our own driveway. But my parents didn't want to see it. It took a transatlantic trip to an obscure country to drive the point home.

In retrospect, even David agreed that the trip to San Marino had been a foolish idea. Not because of what happened, but because of his physical condition. He was still walking laboriously with a cane, but he couldn't hold a book—much less a suitcase —without toppling. Logistically complicated, the trip required weeks of meticulous planning. Since Pauline was leaving a week early to visit her mother in Israel, Dana and Leora and I (now home on vacation) would take David to the airport. A friend in New York would help him change flights, and Pauline would pick him up in a rented car in Rome. The careful design required that the trip be snag-proof: no late planes, no lay-overs. The whole point was to bask in a week of sunshine with all the old friends, physicians, and scientists who would gather in southern Italy for the annual International Endocrine Conference. The burden of responsibility made Pauline think twice, but she knew it might be their last trip together. And David said, "It might be my last chance." He assured her: once they arrived at the conference they would not be alone. There would be hundreds of helping hands. The whole endocrine community, which wrapped itself around the globe like a mammoth fishing net held together by phone calls, overlapping research and conferences, would be there.

The trip was a disaster. Not because the planes were late—they were on time. The Hertz Rent-A-Car was waiting for them in Rome. It was something else. Maybe David should have realized or at least suspected. After all, reports of new developments travel quickly in the scientific community. David knew his colleagues around the world had learned of his illness, either through rumors, direct report, deduction, or independent diagnosis. Only a few individuals had written or called. Of course he noticed— each absence was palpable. Still, he thought, things would be different in person. Face to face. They would see he was the same fellow he'd always been, that he expected no heavy scenes or emotional farewells. He knew why he hadn't heard from his colleagues: they simply didn't know what to say. ALS was a death sentence. Speaking about it would be trespassing onto emotionally volatile ground, sensitive, forbidden, and private. Scientists are trained to deal with data, statistics, test tubes, and Geiger counters. Confronted with this thing—abstract, unmanageable, unmeasurable, and uncontrollable—many were reduced to babbling and stuttering. There was no knowledge within which to contain David's illness. Nothing with which to break it down, explain it, X-ray and diagram it. There were no formulae, no methodology, neither theory nor hypothesis. It was greater than him—greater than all of them—greater than their grants and their computer labs and their bibliographies. Their tools were useless, impotent. And they were terrified. He thought he would pleasantly surprise them by showing up at the conference, but he was wrong. The last thing they expected was to see him, invading their carefully monitored world of proof and conclusions as he stumbled into the convention center, cane in hand.

As soon as David and Pauline walked into the crowded grand ballroom to register their names, they could feel it. For a fraction of a second, the chatter of the crowd dimmed. People turned, stared, and looked away. Then they quickly resumed their conversations, out of discomfort saying anything that came to mind, any words that would fill up space. And then, quietly, in a whisper: He's so sick . . . My goodness . . . What a shock to see him here. As David proceeded toward the registration counter the crowd parted like the Red Sea to make way for him. But it was a gesture of fear more than courtesy. Only a handful of old friends came up to kiss Pauline on the cheek, pat David gently on the back, "Glad you made it." The majority scrambled to safely distant spots. Pauline tried to make a joke of it. "They must think there's plutonium in your cane," she said.

That first day set the tone for the entire convention. People who did not greet them that first day at registration avoided them for three days and nights. They fidgeted when David came near, and stuttered sentence fragments when he tried to start up conversations. When my parents stood on the curb waiting for the bus that was to take them to the lecture halls, the rest of the crowd gathered several feet away. When my parents sat down at the dining hall, old friends would file past them without even saying hello. Late-comers who had no choice but to sit at their table busied themselves with the intricate cutting of their beef

Wellington, then quickly left the cafeteria for their rooms. Only a few of the hundreds of familiar faces sought David out, offered him a hand, made sure he and Pauline didn't eat alone.

"Thank God for Leonard. He's been a real sport," Pauline sighed. "I wonder what's wrong with them—think we should remind them it isn't contagious?"

But David wasn't in the mood for laughter. "Hell, they're doctors. They know."

"Maybe they're confused and they think it's leprosy."

"I'm really sorry to put you through this, Pauline."

"It's not your fault, for Pete's sake. Gosh, even Keith. He must have had dinner at our house in Jerusalem six or seven times. Every time he was in the country I had him over. And Brody— of all people, Brody—he and I have known each other since high school. But we really shouldn't be shocked, should we? We're pretending to be shocked but this isn't really the first time, is it? Right, Dov?"

"I was just about to say that. We can't pretend it's only happening here."

"And there I was thinking it could only happen in Nashville. How naive of me. I thought it was some southern thing," Pauline said. And she thought, being alone in the midst of a crowd has got to be the worst kind of loneliness.

"I don't think I ever believed it was a southern habit. It's a universal human response, unfortunately. I don't think that means it's inevitable."

"Human. Not humane," Pauline said.

But it really was nothing new. If anything, it was déjà vu. Everything that happened here—every incident, each exchange— was just a flashback. Everything reminded them of something else. Like standing on the curb waiting for the limo. Back home, every morning as they pulled up into the special handicapped spot located by the main entrance to the hospital, the doctors making their way to the door scattered. As Pauline and David crossed the lot, Dr. Medweg sat in his car fiddling with the radio dial twenty minutes just to avoid bumping into them. Dr. Carles made a beeline to the door, his eyes looking straight in front of him like a horse. Dr. Salinger had changed his hours: he no longer arrived at the same time they did.

Sitting at the cafeteria restaurant in San Marino, watching friends rush by without a greeting, they had another flashback—to the time Pauline saw her friend Grace at the supermarket. Their eyes met for a split second, and then Grace turned her grocery cart in the opposite direction and scurried away. Grace hadn't wanted to speak with Pauline. If she did, she would have to ask about David. Surely Pauline didn't want to be bothered with that now. It was the wrong time, the wrong place. It was always the wrong time, the wrong place.

Trying to catch Brody's eye as he played with his food was just like trying to catch the eye of a colleague at Vanderbilt, who, upon seeing them, became suddenly engrossed in the mundane pattern of the carpet like a schoolgirl intent on avoiding the cracks in the sidewalk so she wouldn't break her mother's back.

You could tell when someone had just found out it was ALS David suffered from, rather than a bad back. The person's whole demeanor would change. It was like that first time with Cheryl Fitzgerald, Elliot's wife, on the telephone. A pause too long between sentences, an awkwardness. They'd hurry through their lines and drop the phone. Some stopped calling. Or said "no" so quickly when you asked them over for coffee—as if they hadn't even checked their calendar, just did the safest thing. They were scared. They didn't know what to do. David was different now. He was a marked man. He was a time bomb, ticking away. What do you say to a time bomb? "How are you?" What do you say to a woman whose husband is dying? "How are things with the family?" What do you say to a brilliant scientist who knows he is going to die? "How's the research going?" How do you respond to the two people, who, until a few months ago, were the ideal couple. With the beautiful home. Children doing so well. A large circle of friends. It's a crystal bowl with a crack down the middle. You turn it around, so you don't have to look at the crack. Go home, say how tragic it is, how awful and how sad. But to their face, you can't say a thing. You can't think of a thing to say.

As David and Pauline sped away from San Marino in their rented car and headed for a hotel by the sea "wherever we can find some sun," they tried to regain their composure and take stock.

"We have to face this thing head on, and decide on an approach," David said. "All is not lost. It was a terrible experience, but let's try to learn something from it."

"It was terrible—it was a nightmare! I can't imagine three more hellish days," Pauline answered.

"At least it opened our eyes to something that we have stubbornly refused to acknowledge until now. We're going to face this at home, so let's use this time to figure out our strategy."

"But why? Why would people do such a thing?" Pauline cried out. Sometimes David was so cool, so cerebral, she envied him. "I don't understand. They see you struggling to get across the room—don't they see you have enough to contend with already? It's so cruel. My God, they must have known you didn't come all this way just to hear some lousy lectures . . ."

"But look at the people who did make an effort—who really tried to take care of us. And I honestly believe not one person at the conference meant to hurt me. They just didn't know how to approach us. You must realize that, Pauli."

"I realize it on one level, but on another level I don't understand it at all. What does it take to come up to someone, say hello? It's such a simple gesture. That's all I wanted; nothing more complicated than a 'Hello, how are you?' "

"Well, the question now is what we're going to do about it. We have to challenge it, not bow to it. Communication is going to be a key factor."

"We also have really terrific friends back home," Pauline said. "There are some people I trust absolutely and have no qualms about. This thing really separated the wheat from the chaff, didn't it? I just have to keep reminding myself to focus on the wheat instead of on the chaff. . . ."

The wheat: friends like the Bowers. Wayne and Eve had been worried about David since that first June. Both were educators, unfamiliar with the field of medicine, so they didn't know the exact source of the problem. But it was no "back problem"—they had seen bad backs before. They didn't know it was ALS. They didn't have a name for it, but what's in a name? It was bad—they knew that intuitively. More than that, they really didn't want to know. They preferred partial ignorance. That was their denial. So they came over in the evenings, just like they had before, and they discussed the same things they had discussed before—politics, education, a little gossip, and who's divorcing whom. It was a genuine friendship, no trappings needed. Like Pauline and David, they didn't drink; they didn't even like tea or coffee. And there was no need to go out together, to catch a film or a concert. It was enough just to talk, share experiences and ideas. Art, music, work; stories of children and mischief and growing up. Sometimes after they left it seemed everything—almost everything—was right with the world, and good.

The Bowers acknowledged the illness, but didn't focus on it. Other people agonized over whether to invite my parents to a party or not. But the Bowers saw the limp, and then the cane, and they started saying, "When can we come and see you?" instead of "Would you like to come over on Thursday evening?" Eve brought a three-course meal over one evening, because, as she put it, "We wanted to have you over for dinner." And when Pauline called to cancel a date because David was tired, they were not offended. They knew what she was talking about. They had seen David become quiet and weary at the end of an evening. Once when Pauline mentioned that people seemed reluctant to visit, Eve had said, "Gosh, if we don't come for a week or two, we feel something is missing—we just have to come over."

There were other friends as well. People like Susie Warner. Susie was an occupational therapist. Every time she saw David she got an idea for a gadget, an exercise for his limbs, a special pillow for him to sit on. She would go home and return with a sample, and if it worked, she would order one for him through the reams of catalogues and toll-free 800 numbers she collected at the office.

And there was Rona, Dana's music teacher and a wonderful flautist. In between performances with the Nashville Symphony she played in community concerts with a trio of musicians. She knew David was a music lover, and one day she made a suggestion. When she and her trio were preparing for a concert, she said, well, they could use a dress rehearsal in front of a small audience. Our baby grand wasn't getting much exercise these days, she said, and "Y'know what they say, if Muhammad can't go to the mountain." Pauline and David thought it was an excellent idea.

But then there was the chaff. People who had backed off, as if to say, "Oh boy, this is serious stuff. We'll, uh, see you later." Most disappointing were the Kayes. Our "old family friends." At least that's what we used to call them. The Kayes seemed— well, almost angry about David's illness. As if it had been a personal affront to them. As if David had let them down by becoming ill, broke some sort of promise. The friendship became a burden to them. There was no joy left in it for them— they saw only demands, and felt only guilt. Even though all Pauline and David had ever wanted was their continued companionship.

"Some people just aren't up to it, and I guess we have to accept that," David said to her suddenly. They must have been thinking along the same lines and come full circle. "You can't force people to be friends if they don't want to be. What we can do is try to clear the air and work out any communication lapses that may have developed along the way. But many of our friends genuinely enjoy us, and being with them is a real boost to me. It lifts me up. And the family has been terrific. The children are a real joy. That's one thing we really have going for us, and should never take for granted. The six of us are a unit, and always will be.

"So we have to remember: the glass is half empty, but it is also half full."

CHAPTER 7

Dana and Leora

Only when we took Dad to the airport on his way to Italy had I realized that Dana and Leora *knew*. We were planning to see Woody Allen's *Stardust Memories* after we put David on the plane. "Don't get a shock—he mentions my illness," Dad told all of us. "It's just at the beginning of the film. It's no big deal. Mom and I were taken aback so I wanted to warn you. But it's a lovely movie, you'll enjoy it."

At the ticket counter we found out the plane was leaving from gate number 24 so we asked for a wheelchair. They brought out a bright red one with American Airlines printed boldly across the back. It had a high back with an aluminum arch that rose six feet into the air. In it David looked small and frail, dressed up in his three-piece Pierre Cardin suit. He smiled up at us, winked, and told us to take care and drive slowly. Then he left, and all three of us pretended to scratch our foreheads while we dried our eyes inconspicuously with our palms. We could talk about it later.

"It just happened," Dana explained. "They didn't plan to tell us, at least it didn't seem planned. It was at the end of dinner. We had a fight—or more, just frustration at Dad's condition. And Mom and Dad said, now don't go look up ALS because it'll just upset you."

"Yeah, and I was really mad 'cause it took me forever to find

out what it stood for so I could look it up in the encyclopedia,"
Leora said. "When we went to that movie I kept saying it over and
over again so I wouldn't forget it, but I still forgot it."

"Maybe I was naive because I didn't realize he was going to
duh," Dana said.

"What?" Leora demanded.

"Die. Die, okay?"

"Well, you have to face up to reality!" Leora said, severely.

"She gets mad when I don't say it," Dana explained to me.

That was Dana for you: when unpleasant subjects came up
she'd say, "I don't want to talk about it," and run out of the room.
Her idea of the ideal summer job was to work in a Hallmark
card store, with the pink racks and Fannie May candies on a
lazy susan, all the grief neatly contained in gilded condolence
cards.

"Anyway it took me about two weeks and then I realized,"
Dana said. "By the time we went to *Stardust Memories* I'm sure
I knew. There was something before that too. Mom said, 'Well
you are going through something different. You're watching your
father become paralyzed.' That was a long time ago, in ninth
grade. I asked her why he didn't get an operation and she said,
'There is no operation.' But back then I didn't think he was
going to die. I asked her, could Daddy die from it? And she said
yes . . . but I thought it was an outside chance. I was suspicious
before because she was being such a mother hen to Daddy, saying
eat, eat! That was in the summer when he had just started walking
with a limp. But he was doing so much exercise, and you know we
were brought up that if you do exercise you're healthy so I thought
he must be healthy. I remember that one afternoon. Mom said
to Dad, walk up the hill. And she watched him. And I said, you
better go to a doctor, Dad. And I got really mad at him."

"I didn't buy that disk story for one second," Leora said. "But
I didn't realize he was going to die either. I thought he'd be a
quadraplegic and just have his head. I wanted to look ALS up
but I didn't know what it stood for. I asked my biology teacher
but just so it wouldn't look suspicious I made a list of abbrevia-
tions: VD, MS, MD, all this stuff. Until then I thought . . . no,
it's really silly I won't tell you. . . ."

Leora looks tough, but one day after that time at the airport I walked into her room and found her sitting on the bed, red-faced and crying. "Don't you dare walk in here without knocking!" she said fiercely, regaining her composure. "And when I'm not here either. Don't you dare walk in here!" "Okay, okay," I said, retreating. And from behind the door I whispered, "Are you okay?" But she didn't answer.

"In all my dreams Dad is healthy," Leora said. "And I say all right, Dad! You're walking without your cane! And he says, sure kiddo. And he's always doing things, playing tennis, or just walking. In one dream, I remember, he was walking next to Mom, without his cane. I thought he must be leaning on her but he wasn't.

"God," she said, "I feel so bad. I used to race him when we went swimming and I'd say, hey, either you're getting slower or I'm getting faster. And he'd say, no, I'm just getting old."

That's strange, because generally Leora is intuitive about Dad's needs, coming up with an arm or a chair just when he needs it. Usually it is Dana who hesitates, unsure, scared she will do the wrong thing at the wrong time.

"I was never mad at them for not telling me sooner," Dana said emphatically, as if to clear the air. "Never. I was grateful. Always."

"Did you tell your friends?" I asked. "I only told three friends at Oberlin: Eve, Brett, and Bill. Later I told Regina and Connie. But I was mad at myself—I didn't want to become 'girl with dying father.' And it seemed like the greater the number of people who didn't know—and had no reason to suspect—the more normal I was, the more I could pull it off."

"Some of my friends are real bitches when it comes to Dad," Leora said in her unambiguous way. "They never ask me how he is. Not Carrie; not Sally; not Melanie; not Beverly. I always ask Carrie how her family is, and I ask Sally how she's doing. And I always say, in a joke sort of, but serious, "If you ever want to talk I can be your psychiatrist." They never—never!—ask me. Everybody's a jackass in this world. Bob asks me sometimes. Melanie says, 'Gosh I don't know what I'd do if my father even got a cold.' But she never asks either. I told Melissa and she just spread it around a little bit. Sweet Melissa."

"I hate all my friends," Dana said. "I'm sorry, it's the truth. Except for Harriet and Corinne. I hate everyone else. Especially Vicky and Leslie and Tina. . . ."

"Well, all those people's parents dropped us, so what do you expect? Their parents all dropped Mom and Dad," Leora said.

"But they were over here for dinner a couple of months ago," Dana said. "And they saw. They saw how Daddy was. And I know that when he dies they'll come up to me and say they're so sorry and be so nice. It just makes me sick. I dread that day. I'll be so upset already and I'll have to put up with their hypocrisy."

"Well, just say, 'Look, you guys, you weren't supportive to me while my father was sick so I'd rather not be with you now, I'd rather be with people who were supportive,' " I said.

"I think potheads are better friends," Leora said. "No, seriously, Dana, don't shake your head at me like that."

"That is so stupid, Leora," Dana said.

"No. 'Cause lots of times they've had all kinds of problems, so they're more sensitive," Leora tried to explain. "And they're into psychology and stuff. Most people really don't think it's such a big deal what we're going through. I really think they don't. They just think it's something about you."

"But death is different," Dana argued. "Death is different from dying. That's why I'm so scared about that day. I'm scared that people won't know, and will come up and ask me and I'll break down. Or they will know and won't say anything."

"It's so incredible. I can't believe it really will happen," Leora said. "That a day will come and he won't be here anymore. And then he never will again. I always think he'll be there in his chair, in that corner of the room. . . ."

"In a way we're all just waiting, waiting for that day to happen and hoping it won't happen . . . like Mom says, it's a twilight war," Dana said.

"Leora, didn't you have a big fight with your advisor?" I asked. "What was that all about?"

"Wait, wait," Dana interrupted. "First I want to put in a good word about advisors—before she says anything. Mr. White has been really nice to me. I don't know how he knew. I guess everyone knows—"

"*Everyone* knows, Dana," Leora said, unequivocally.

"Okay. But that's okay. I think it's important for the teacher to know, even though I don't let it affect my performance and I don't think it should be used as an excuse. I think they should be told things like that."

Dana gets straight A's. It comes easily to her; she's disciplined and she can sit. Practices her flute for half an hour every day. Leora's hyper; she has to buckle down. I think she does it mostly for Dad. Last report card she brought home was straight A's in all but Phys Ed—I guess she skipped too many times, running down to the Quik Sak with her friends, to buy candy and hang out.

Dana went on. "Anyway, Mr. White called me into his office to talk about it. And he's been consistent—he always asks how Daddy is and how we are and everything."

"I don't know, Dan," Leora said. "I got really upset with him when he taught the course on Death and Dying. When he said that he thought it was better to go through the five stages than to die instantly in your sleep. I didn't even want to listen to that."

"He must have lost someone very suddenly, Lok," I interjected. "And he probably felt it would have been better to have a chance to tell the person certain things that he never got around to."

"Yeah, I think he did," Dana answered. "I didn't like that course either, Leora. Five stages—makes it sound so neat and simple, one-two-three. And that just isn't true. You can't explain it. You feel everything at once. I accept death, but in a way I can't believe it. And I'm angry at my friends, all the time. Mr. White and I talked about that. We're worried about me hating people. . . ." Her voice trailed off.

"I guess I'm worried too. For all of us," I said.

"Okay, you better listen," Leora said. "This is the story about my advisor. I don't know why, but one day I told her about Dad. I was really upset, especially about my friends because they didn't seem to care and never asked and everything. So I talked to her once, and then when she ran into Mom she told her what I had told her. I was so mad. I went up to her and said she was unconfidential—in these words—unconfidential, immoral, and unethical. I told her I knew she hadn't had any guidance training except as a human being; I had told her those things in confidence and I thought she would respect that. And I told her, that even though I had explained that what bothered me about my friends was that they never asked, she never asked either. Anyway she got super-upset. I kind of felt sorry for her. She said that she always wanted to ask me but I was always surrounded by a crowd of people. I said, you could pull me aside. She got so upset; she started crying and everything. I said, sorry, I didn't mean to upset you. She's a lot better now; she's really nice to me."

"She's probably scared of you," I said, not entirely joking.

"Don't you ever wonder sometimes what we'd be doing if Dad wasn't sick?" Leora asked. "We'd probably go camping a lot; we used to go camping a whole lot. We'd probably go to Sefton's wedding in South Africa, and to the World's Fair in Knoxville. . . . But y'know what scares me the most? When I think that something could happen to another one of us. That one of us would get sick, or be in a car accident. That would kill me, it would totally kill me. If it had to happen again I'd rather it happen to me. Just so I don't have to go through this again. I couldn't. I just couldn't. It's selfish, but I'd rather it happen to me."

"I wonder what'll happen to Mom when Dad dies," I whispered.

"I know," Dana said, "she'll force herself to comfort us for a while, then—poof!"

"I always worry that the person I marry should know Daddy," Dana said. "He's such an influence on me, on all of us. It seems like in order for someone to understand me, he'd have to know Daddy. And I want to have a family like ours. It's special. We do things together and we stick together. My friend Vicky's family doesn't even eat dinner together."

"God? I never believed in God." Dana doesn't say it frivolously; she's given it a lot of thought. She had long conversations with the rabbi in her confirmation classes. "I hate God. And I decided it wasn't even an issue of whether there is a God or not, but whether I believe in Him or not. And I don't. Even if there is, in reality, a God, I don't believe in Him."

Then Dana asked Leora to tell me something, but Leora hesitated.

"No, it's stupid . . . it's so embarrassing. . . ."

"C'mon—we won't laugh, I promise," I told her.

Finally, after much prodding, Leora opened up.

"Well, . . . no, it's . . . Okay, I'll tell you. I thought you had this disease for ten years and became a quadraplegic and then—then, if you went to the beach, like we did, at Hilton Head . . . if you went to the beach, you got better. And there's another part. If relatives came. If relatives came and you went to the beach."

And I realized: we had all believed that, that summer.

CHAPTER 8

A New Routine

Back in the United States David said it was the craziest thing he'd ever done. Not only that, but what kind of vacation could it have been for Pauline, traveling around with a sick man, trying to find barrier-free hotels in southern Italy? When they landed back in Kennedy she had put him on a plane to D.C., where their good friends Al and Evelyn picked him up. He stayed at their house while he participated in an NIH study section. "It may be your last one," Pauline said gently. "Call me every day. Are you sure you can manage?"

In Washington Dad rented a walker, a three-dimensional stainless steel stick with an option to buy. Al and Evelyn were great— they always were. Al had voted for Reagan, and David grilled him about it. Evelyn was a painter; she showed David her latest, beige and light blue, lots of sunshine. David told them the funniest thing had happened in New York: they were taking a cab from Kennedy to La Guardia. Pauline had run off for a minute and he had stumbled into the cab, leaving the bag with the passports and traveler's cheques on the sidewalk. When Pauline got into the cab she said in Hebrew: *"Tipesh! Hisharta et hatik!"* meaning: "Stupid! You left the bag." The cab driver turned around. *"Ein sodot poh,"* he said in Hebrew. "No secrets here, lady!"

If I can just make it through this winter, David thought. It was time to change things, get into a routine, do what he had always said: develop an alternative lifestyle, balance hope and realism, temper optimism with pragmatism. He'd lost a week of swimming in Italy; he couldn't afford that any more. He had to get his priorities straight. Work at home two days a week, rest every afternoon, be more efficient. Just to make it through the winter. He made a plan:

Don't go to rounds every day.

Come home early (two-thirty). Have some lunch and sleep for a couple of hours. Then swim.

Alternate days: bike 1½ miles on stationary bike.

Lots of sleep at night.

No more traveling. Maybe spend next winter in South Africa. Something to look forward to, anyway.

Strict regimen. The only exception: fatigue.

Diet: Aim for 70–100 grams of protein a day. Healthy people can afford to be flexible and take a lot of protein one day, little or none the next, and the body balances itself out. Nature is very versatile. Can't take for granted the diseased body will do the same, especially in a muscle-wasting disease.

Everything took longer now: the walk from the bedroom to the bathroom, the hike from the bathroom to the kitchen. David had a ritual he went through in the morning: sitting on the side of the bed he pulled one foot up until it rested on the opposite knee, fitted a sock on, lassoed one trouser leg onto his foot, shoved it back on the floor. Now the other side: pull, fit, lasso, shove. Then a battle with each shoe, crossing the leg over again, attaching the bootie—it's easy, attaches with Velcro—then shove. Velcro on the trousers instead of buttons—Velcro pastes on and off, great stuff. Laces, buttons, zippers, clasps, ties, bows—tiny, delicate, intricate mechanisms he couldn't handle anymore. He bought his shirts loose now, turtle-necks mostly—they were the easiest, sporty but acceptable at the hospital, didn't choke around the neck like the button-downs, and made the lack of a tie less glaring. And no buttons.

Then it was time to confront the bathroom. First he had to get there. Station himself in front of the sink. Get the walker out of the way. Lean forward to get balanced. Start the ritual. First a face cloth, easier to wash with than partially paralyzed hands. Then he would shave with a light disposable razor. The first time he used the disposable razor instead of his regular razor he thought he was getting better. It was so light! Then he realized the disposable razor weighed less than two ounces. . . . Shave the right side with the right hand, then the left with the left. Then the teeth: unscrew the cap of the toothpaste, coordinate the mouth of the tube with the brush, spread the right amount, recap the tube. It was Pauline's idea to use an electric toothbrush. His hands couldn't make sharp little up-and-down motions anymore, and he had been getting a crick in his neck from shaking his head back and forth.

The morning consisted of a series of steps, each one relying on the completion of the one before it, and futile unless the one after it was successful. He had to concentrate. The slightest disturbance could ruin the whole chain. An unexpected yell, a knock at the door, Leora stomping her feet in adolescent rage over the inadequacy of her wardrobe. These things could drive him crazy in the mornings.

One day Dana knocked at the door while he was dressing. His left leg, pulled but not yet lassoed or shoved into his pants, fell to the floor. Damn it, he had to start all over again.

"Do you have any trash?" she asked.

"Go away. I'm dressing."

Two days later it happened again, "Trashwoman here." David blew up. Didn't he tell her? Only in case of an emergency was she to knock in the mornings. Poor Dana was frightened and ran away. "Come back here," David called to her. As he tried to explain: the morning is the hardest time for him, he's at his crabbiest, he's vulnerable. Getting dressed is so difficult, the hardest, after that the rest of the day is a snap.

"Okay, I understand. But I just wanted to help. I didn't mean to get in the way," Dana said, pouting. She was so sensitive to his criticism that he hesitated to say anything. And sometimes he had to remind her: just because he's sick doesn't mean he's always right, doesn't mean they can't disagree. But she was scared—scared she was not helping enough, not helping the right way. Scared he'd get mad at them and go away. Go away mad, or go away earlier than he had to.

Over breakfast a news article caught David's eye.

It was one of an increasing number of pieces attempting to pinpoint and analyze the questions surrounding the right to die issue. Is life by grace of medical technology really life? In the case of a mentally incompetent patient, who is to play God? Most doctors won't—they don't want to be sued. Should families? Do they have the right and the necessary knowledge? Several states were trying to draw up guidelines for families in this predicament. The article that morning described a court ruling that made a distinction between those patients who made clear before becoming unconscious that they had no desire to live in a state of vegetative coma, and those who had not. If a patient with no chance of recovery had previously stated that he did not want his life artificially maintained, a guardian would be permitted to withdraw life supporting equipment.

David clipped the article out and slipped it into the manila folder he was taking in to work. He had postponed the decision long enough—today he would call his lawyer and draw up a living will. It would be brief and simple, stating that he did not want his life artificially sustained by a respirator. When he was no longer able to breathe on his own, that's the end. No iron lung. Quality, not quantity. When he can't breathe any longer, that's it. There was no hope for recovery in this illness, and what's the point in lingering an extra two or three months?

He'd had this in mind for several months already, but it was very threatening, much more threatening than writing a last will and testament. But now that the textbook was out to the printers, the last check to Oberlin signed with a shaky hand, the papers in order . . . he could do it. He could imagine living after losing the ability to swallow (they can feed you through a tube), or without the faculty of speech (the one set of muscles rarely affected by ALS is that of the eyes, and he could communicate with his family in Morse code), but he didn't want to stick around, tied up to the machine, while the family waited. Without a legal document even the most empathetic physician is obligated to do all he can to keep his patient alive. Euthanasia is against the law and the physician can be prosecuted for murder. And once the patient is unconscious or unable to communicate he has no control. So while he was still able, David wanted to make sure there was a document which would "clearly and convincingly show" that he didn't want to "be maintained . . . by use of a respirator."

CHAPTER 9

Teamwork

Just as my father was still "the king" when he walked in the front door at home, he was still the chief at the endocrine division at Vanderbilt. And that was a good thing. He set his long-term goal—"to live until Leora graduates from high school"—by us; he set his short-term goals—up every morning at seven, rain or shine—by the work at the hospital. We nourished him and loved him; the people in his division stimulated him intellectually and respected him. He was lame, but he was still the chief.

The fourth floor of the hospital, which housed the division, was cozy and warm. When David stumbled to the restroom, he always knew he could count on someone seeing him and rushing to hold the door open. His loyal secretary always thought to bring him a cup of coffee or juice—though he never asked it of her. His postgraduate Fellows accompanied him on his long sojourns down the halls, and on good days, when he could walk and talk at the same time, he taught them as he went, referring to articles they should look up ("April or May, 71, in the *British Medical Journal*") or interesting cases he had seen way back ("fascinating case we saw at Hopkins"). He was an encyclopedia full of knowledge. And when he had bad days, they walked slowly, watching his feet and kidding him about his resemblance to Jerry Ford.

Outside of the four endocrinology halls, David never knew what to expect. One day, as he was trudging down the hall concentrating on lifting his walker and throwing his legs in front of him, a voice interrupted his thoughts.

"Still insist on not using a wheelchair, eh?" a condescending voice said. David looked up and saw one of the staff surgeons.

"No, I'm using my walker," he answered.

"What is it, embarrassment, that you don't want to use a wheelchair?"

"No, I'm not embarrassed. I'm very cerebral about my illness. I want to keep using my muscles as long as I can. I use a wheelchair when I have to—I often do, in fact, in airports and museums. But I use it only if I have to, and I'm very good at deciding what is and isn't fatiguing for me."

"Well, it's amazing that an endocrinologist can be cerebral. Just a little joke. You're sorry that you ran into me now, aren't you?"

"No, I'm not. I can talk about the illness rationally without becoming emotional. If you want to talk, by all means. I'm not embarrassed by the conversation."

"Oh, good. Well, see you, David." And then the surgeon had hurried off in the opposite direction, leaving David to continue his slow, long walk to his office. David lifted the walker, pushed it forward, took a step. He felt hurt, and he could hardly believe what had happened. The man had stopped him, gibed at him for his struggle instead of encouraging him, and then run off without a care in the world.

Several months ago, when David was still walking with the cane, he had fallen in front of the hospital. For a few moments he lay on the ground, unable to move a muscle. Then a physician walked by. Help is on the way, David thought. He managed to catch the doctor's eye and waited for him to approach. But the doctor quickly looked away, pretending not to see David lying in the middle of the parking lot. Before David knew it, his colleague had disappeared into a doorway and was gone. As he lay there, waiting for someone to come to his aid, he said to himself, "I can't get upset about it. I have to keep my cool. It's the illness they're reacting to, not me. I must be cerebral. It's not worth getting emotional about."

By December David was accustomed to reactions of this sort, so George Wirth's offer to swim with him came as a complete surprise. Dr. Wirth was an endocrinologist who had joined the staff at Vanderbilt after training as a fellow. He was a young man, about thirty years old, quiet and thoughtful. He had been through a brief, unhappy marriage a year earlier, and David had been very helpful to him in the months that followed.

"I swim every day anyway," he told David. "And you really shouldn't be out there alone, or even with Dana and Leora. What if you get a cramp? They can't pull you out on their own." It was true; David was like dead weight off his feet.

"That's very generous of you, George," David said. "Of course, it would be a tremendous help, and it would reduce a lot of anxiety. Let's try to work around your schedule and try to find a time that's convenient for you. I don't want to interfere with your other responsibilities."

George became David's coach, and like a coach, he was persistent and demanding. Every day he gave David a ride home from Vanderbilt. He picked David up in his office and walked with him and his walker to the elevator, where he held the doors open as David carefully climbed over the gratings that most people don't even notice. George had the patience of a Buddha. He brought his car around and helped David in; then, at our house he waited while David went through the arduous process of dressing and undressing. Then they set out through the back door, down the three steps, onto the smooth gravel driveway, across the small parking lot, on to Lois's grassy yard, through sticks and stones and roots and acorns and twigs that can trip. At the pool George had to fold David through the three-foot-high entrance to the bubble, and then lower him carefully into the water. An hour later they would emerge from the pool, sopping wet. Luckily it was a mild winter; even so, it was cold, and if Dana or Leora were home from school they would run out to replace George so he could get back inside and warm up. The walk from one yard to the other could take David twenty minutes—just luck that he didn't catch pneumonia. Some days he was so exhausted by the time he got back inside that George had to help him dress. By the time they were done it was time for the evening news, the girls were bustling around in the kitchen preparing lots of protein, and Pauline would invite George to stay for dinner. George was stubborn: if David ever felt like skipping a day he talked him out of it. And when the disease had progressed to the point that just putting on his bathing suit exhausted David, George dressed him so the precious energy could be used for swimming. He had to keep those muscles moving.

When George offered to move in so that he could be closer and able to help David on a daily basis, we were even more surprised. So many friends had turned their backs—and here was someone coming forth with an offer much more considerate and generous than we could imagine, much less expect. There was no question that George would be of great help in the months ahead. Already it took more than a simple shove to pull David up from a chair. Or the car. Or the bed.

"All those things are much easier for me than for you because I'm stronger," George told Pauline. "If I lived with you I could drive David in to work and bring him home every day."

"You could do that without actually moving in, though," Pauline answered. "Maybe things will get to a point where we'll have to have someone come in but right now we can manage. Don't you see?—once you move in it's an all-the-time thing, twenty-four hours a day. It's terribly draining. Even when you go out it's on your mind, and you have to return to it. It's very stressful. You may not realize what a huge commitment it is. How it engulfs your whole life, even if you set limits on it."

"But I don't want to set limits. That's exactly it. If I live here I can be totally committed. I won't leave. It wouldn't be a temporary thing. I'm not going to leave. I would only leave if my parents needed me."

"But George—that's crazy! You can't give up the rest of your life. You're a young guy. What if David lives for another five or ten years?"

"But I don't see it as giving up anything. I can go on living my normal life here. I enjoy being with David; I enjoy helping him. He's so vibrant. I learn from him all the time. It's not painful or strenuous for me to spend time with him. On the contrary. It's a treat."

"What about your personal and social life?"

"They don't play such a big role for me. . . . Listen. The last thing I want is to intrude at a time like this. I know your family needs a lot of time alone together. I understand that, so I think you should discuss it with them. But I really care for David and I'd like to help."

The family voted yes—"whatever's best for Daddy." The sunroom would have to be converted into a bedroom . . . we'd have to clear out a chest of drawers for George, and a book shelf. . . .

"We're very grateful to you for this, George; I don't know how we can ever thank you," Pauline said.

"Don't thank me," he answered. "I enjoy it. I'm doing it for purely selfish reasons."

"Well, I can't really believe that. Anyway, it takes a lot of stress off the family. Just knowing someone's here. I can't tell you. But we can't have this never-leave stuff; it isn't fair to you. You have no way of gauging how you'll feel six months from now. We should have an evaluation every six months—or sooner. You should never feel you have to stay. It's a tremendous thing you're doing; you don't realize."

"Well, I'm not going to leave unless you ask me to. I've told the children that as well."

At the end of January George moved in and joined the team. We all adhered to David's philosophy: there was a logical solution to any problem, given a calm and rational approach. ALS wasn't pleasant, you wouldn't wish it on your enemies, but it wasn't necessarily a death sentence either; you could learn to live with it. David was still telling people who called long-distance to ask how he was, that he was "just having some difficulties getting around," or "having problems with my legs." Every day there was a new problem to solve. David and George figured out a "system" for everything: a system for getting David to work, a system for getting him out of the pool. In addition to the swimming, George did passive exercises with David, which helped prevent his arms and legs from freezing at the shoulder, hip, and knee joints. We got a bath chair with a hydraulic pump to raise and lower Dad into the bath, and found that a lightweight hair dryer was an easy way for him to dry himself. With it he could reach the tough spots around the groin and underarms, thus avoiding the fungal infections patients with neurological illnesses are prone to, as well as maintaining a much appreciated, albeit minor, measure of independence.

He was also reconsidering his attitude toward experimental drugs. Earlier, David had scoffed at drugs that had been proven ineffectual by what he considered careful and methodical studies. He saw no need to try them out himself. He applied to them the same principles that he adhered to in his own research, even in his tests with lecithin—if a drug was effective it would be effective in a small group of subjects and in a single study, without the need for continuous and repetitious studies involving hundreds of subjects. He hadn't changed his mind about this, but two additional factors entered into his consideration. First, he realized that the insidious "creeping" nature of the disease, as well as the variation between individuals, made it very difficult to produce clear and definitive results, even in the best of studies. Secondly, he realized that his illness was progressing defiantly, in spite of his exercise program and disciplined efforts. It was getting to the point where he was willing to try almost anything to stop it. Doctors had tried all sorts of modalities on ALS patients: plasmapheresis, vitamin E, guanidine (a substance that acts like acetylcholine), mestinol (which destroys the enzyme that destroys acetylcholine), and baclofen (an analogue of a natural neurotransmitter, thought to dampen the anterior horn cells, or lower motor neurons). Vitamin E and guanidine weren't thought to be effective. Baclofen produced unpleasant side effects: loss of balance, and dizziness. Mestinol caused cramping, diarrhea, changes in visual ability and focus, an increase in the amount of fasciculation. Fasciculation was a topic of debate in the medical world. No one really knew whether muscle twitching was a sign of dying muscle or whether it signified the body's attempt to rebuild the muscle. One thing was certain: it was very uncomfortable. Considering that these drugs had no definite positive effects, David saw no point in subjecting himself to them.

There were two other choices. One was interferon, an anti-viral substance that the body normally makes when invaded by a virus. It had been used effectively in some cancer patients, and if ALS was caused by a sort of virus it might be helpful. Interferon is difficult to obtain since it is very expensive to isolate. Even in the purest form available only one percent of the solution is pure interferon. With his contacts in the medical world it was conceivable that David might be able to get hold of some, but he decided against it. In a six-month comparison study of a group of treated ALS patients and a control group, results showed severe side effects and no benefits.

Then there was levamisol, which stimulates a portion of the immune system. If the immune theory for ALS was true, then the drug might be potentially useful. So far there was no evidence in favor of the drug, but no significant evidence to the contrary either. So David decided to try it. It produced no harmful side effects and it couldn't hurt, so why not?

David's ideas about experimental drugs were really very simple. Just common sense really. If a drug were hailed as having a therapeutic effect, the patient should by all means try it. But if there were no scientific evidence to back up the claims, and yet the drug had indisputable negative side effects, such as discomfort or nausea, well, ultimately it was up to the patient. For some, the psychological comfort derived from knowing one is taking a drug—any drug at all—may override the discomfort. But again, that should always be the patient's choice. Most scientists would probably agree that it would be naive to apply the concept of the placebo effect to all diseases, particularly terminal illness.

David was still taking Valium regularly, but Valium is only a symptomatic medication. In other words, it relieves the symptoms by reducing spasticity, but it doesn't get at the causes of the illness. He took it only at night; ten milligrams reduced the twitching and spasm and gave him a good seven hours of sleep. But since Valium is addictive, he stayed away from it during the day unless he was very stiff. ALS produces both spasticity and weakness. There may be an advantage to the spasticity, because when the muscles are tight (spastic) the weakness is reduced. In other words, the spasm may in fact be a bonus, enabling the patient to walk and function.

For a while David thought he was improving. At least, stabilizing. He attributed it to the passive exercises, the levamisol, the regulation of his routine. (He took levamisol for a full year, before deciding it wasn't doing anything.) He was writing with great difficulty, but he said he had regained some movement in his left thumb. He said he was lifting his legs whereas before he had been dragging them. And he had a new routine: he took walks down the driveway to the mailbox. Twice daily on days he wasn't swimming.

A few weeks later David had a sudden bout of weakness—a whole new crop of cells had died. Sure, he had thought, I can live without my legs. Still read, write, enjoy the sunshine, watch a play, listen to Beethoven. But why this sudden drop?

"That's the nature of your disease," Fitzgerald said, "to get weaker all the time. It's progressive. You know that."

"But I was doing so well. I want you to run some tests."

"I don't know what tests I can run that will tell you anything."

Sure, he had thought, he could live without the use of his arms: could still read, enjoy the sunshine, watch a play, listen to Beethoven. He ran some tests himself and found that his potassium levels were very low. Aha! So that's what it was. He started supplementing his bodily potassium with an artificial mixture called "K-Lyte." (He eventually stopped when eating became a problem.) In the meantime, potassium became the new lecithin, the placebo, the miracle drug.

And he said sure, he could live without his arms and his legs. As long as he could still communicate with the people he loves. Enjoy the sunshine, listen to Beethoven. And he proceeded to tell us about an article in *The New Republic*, and how his work on the male contraceptive might yield a treatment for cancer of the testis. He told us we shouldn't be bitter—if anything, he was amazed at the number of people who have pulled through and supported us and kept on coming. And if there's one thing he wants to leave us with it's not bitterness but hope and the love of life he's always had. That's what he's fighting for; we should remember that.

From his desk he made phone calls, dictated letters straight onto his secretary's tape at Vanderbilt, controlled the world. He reeled sentences off the top of his head; they would be typed and ready to go the next day.

And he said, sure, he can live like this; still read, listen to Beethoven, communicate with his family. But we watched for twitching in his voice box. Mom said she saw a muscle jump at the base of his neck. Our eyes were glued.

PART **3**

From My Journal

September 1981

I've come back home. After graduation, my friends went on to wait tables in New York City, work for Greenpeace, take a year off and apply to law school, join rock 'n' roll bands. I ran around this summer, but I've decided my place is here in Nashville right now. Dad and I will start working on this book right away. I'm so scared he'll lose his voice before giving me a chance to put his words down on paper; scared he'll leave before telling his story.

My father is dying.

I pretend he isn't. We all pretend he isn't. He makes this easy. "Listen, chump," he says to his insurance agent on the phone, "get this done PDQ and call me back before five."

George Wirth left this past weekend. He was offered a job on the West Coast near his family, and we encouraged him to take it. He was hesitant—he didn't want to feel he had let us down—but he has to go on with his life. I think he'll be much happier out there. He was never too crazy about Nashville. I must say though, I don't know how we'll manage without him (of course I'd never tell him that). For eight months he was at Dad's beck and call, twenty-four hours a day. It was only thanks to him that David was able to continue going in to work for as long as he did—and his work is so important to him.

143

The question is: What are we going to do now? Dad is much weaker. He's still walking with the walker, but his arms are stiff, and willpower, not nerves, moves his muscles. His voice is low and thick, like a 45 record on 33, and soon it will affect his swallowing. He probably won't be able to swim—we can't possibly get him in and out of the pool alone. It's more of a psychological loss than a physical one at this point, though there's no way of telling what good it may have done. But his combination breast-free-style stroke has degenerated into a straggling doggy paddle. We can try to substitute some breathing exercises and passive exercises. No idea how we'll bathe him.

Main thing is to keep the news from Michael as long as possible. He's just started at Harvard Business School and I'm sure he's nervous. Dad won't hear of his coming home, and I'm sure he'll want to when he hears that George left. Luckily I have some courses to complete for my BA; I'll be able to stay at home with Dad and work on the book.

I keep thinking of what Mom said once: "The worst is yet to come."

September 18

Finally found someone to come in and bathe Dad. Great guy, Willis Williams, a tall man with two arms strong as tree trunks and the most gentle face, who worked over at Vanderbilt for forty-five years as a nursing aide. Willis is great, shows up every Monday, Wednesday, Friday, no fail. Comes in and says to Dad, "Hey, wanna wrestle?" Dad says, "How are you doing?" "Not bad for a young man my age," Willis answers. He's seventy-two. He tells Dad about his eleven children, three of whom are ministers, and about all the doctors he knows in Nashville. "On to the races!" he bellows, as Dad stumbles to the bathroom on his walker. After the bath he gives Dad a rub-down with too much aftershave. Laughs. "Bring on the women and the dancing girls!" When he leaves he cautions Dad: "Y'all stay out of meanness now."

As far as getting reimbursed for the expense by our medical insurance, forget it. It's a no-win situation. They'll only pay if a skilled professional comes in, and then only fifty percent. A

registered nurse hired through a private home care agency costs
twenty-five dollars an hour, and they want to send two people in
order to lift Dad. We don't need an RN though—we just need a
strong man with some experience. In fact, as it turns out, an
RN can't help us. An RN won't bathe someone on his own, and
would need a bring a physical therapist along with him. So we'd
be paying fifty percent times two professionals times eight hours
a day times three days a week times twenty-five dollars an
hour. . . . . It's a Catch-22. We're better off getting a non-
professional and paying for it ourselves. But where the hell do
you find someone like that? Well, we called the hospice, whose
purported main goal is to keep the terminally ill at home, and
they didn't even have any ideas. They suggested we ask Fitzgerald.
Fitzgerald suggested trying the public health department, who
suggested inquiring with the private home care agencies, look
them up in the yellow pages. . . . We found Mr. Williams through
a friend who's a physician. Lucky.

On Tuesdays and Thursdays I get Dad up. I wake up at seven;
by seven-thirty I'm dressed and showered and I go downstairs.
I hate getting him up so early but he insists; some days he'll take
it easy and sleep in until eight. There's an art to raising him off
the bed. Press HEAD UP on the electric bed. Put on his socks,
trousers, open-toed slippers so his toes don't get clawed up. Move
his legs over to the side of the bed—careful not to slide his behind
off. He laughs, but it's dangerous so I pretend to be severe. Hey,
cut it out. Now a shove up, a pull, bring the walker over and
upsy-daisy. While he walks the four yards to the bathroom I
make the bed, turn the radio off, open the curtains, pass him in
the corridor, prepare his toothbrush, a glass of water with a straw,
lay the pills out. . . .
Dana does Saturday, Leora Sunday. Mom does most of the
bedtimes. The days are planned out carefully to avoid excessive
labor. Dad works at the table in the dining room in the mornings.
A short trip to the bathroom at one; then he naps in the big
chair with the lift that sits in the den. Dana and Leora gather in
the den after school; when Mom comes home we have tea in
there, sometimes dinner, and a movie on cable or ARTS. He has

incredible intellectual stamina—he helps Leora with her geometry, then calls Dana in for her chemistry problems, then "You're next, Roni, come in here with that chapter and let's look it over." Once a week there is a lab meeting for the male contraceptive project; other days doctors come to consult about unusual cases, patients with complications, advice on their papers and grants.

September 25
Strange things keep happening with our friends here. A friend of Mom's comes by to return a book. She pulls in the driveway and gets out of her car just as Dad is making his slow, arduous way down to the road—part of his exercise routine. Dad looks up at her and forces a smile and a wink. She looks at him, dazed; then she looks right past him. She comes up to the front door without even saying hello to him. And he continues his long, hard walk. An insignificant domestic interaction turns into major trauma.

Or this: A friend of Dana and Leora's comes home from school with them. Her father will be by to pick her up at six. Ordinarily he would come in to chat with David, ask about the family. But no: he pulls up the driveway and honks. Like a cheap date. His daughter rushes around frantically to collect her books, scarf, mittens.

I don't know what to make of it. But these incidents shock us, like ice-cold bath water. They bear down on us, scrape at us like rough sandpaper, leaving flakes of residue that fall off and leave us diminished, smaller, fragile.

Dad says not to get discouraged. Focus on the positive, he says. And actually, he says, he is surprised at how many good consistent friends we have, at how many people have come through for us. He tells me a story:
At first, he had been very upset by Dr. Fleming's response—or the lack of any. David just assumed he had figured out what the situation was—Fleming was a physician and a colleague, after all. Why was he so cool, his mannerism so offhanded? It turned out Fleming didn't know. He hadn't seen it. He hadn't wanted to see it. This was back when David was still walking with a cane.

Fleming knew David was walking badly, but that was all. He just assumed it was a dislocated disk—a bad back; no big deal; no great catastrophe; nothing to get worked up about. He was shocked when David told him the real cause of his limp. "My God," he said. "My goodness. I didn't realize . . . how serious . . . I'm so sorry. I'm shocked. I'm a little embarrassed, to tell you the truth. Look at me, I've been so into myself, so self-involved. My focus has been totally inward. I haven't had my eyes open to anything outside of myself.

"But listen, David, however inappropriate my behavior has been so far, it'll change, I assure you. I want to be part of this with you. We're going to go through this together, David. Elaine and I, we're going to help you through this. We're going to fight the illness alongside you. You're not going to be alone in this fight. It's going to be our fight too."

I didn't know this story for a long time. Because the Flemings have taken us under their wing since then. Our self-appointed guardian angels. They visit and call. When Elaine goes to the supermarket, she calls, "Y'all need some groceries?" At Baskin-Robbins 31 flavors she picks up a milkshake for Dad and runs it by on her way home. Or she brings a casserole by for dinner, one less thing on Pauli's mind. And she always reminds us: she's available. For rides. Or just a chat on the phone.

But then there are the Kayes—talk about a study in opposites. The Kayes. Our nemesis, if there is such a thing. They had known Mom and Dad since the old Baltimore days when Dad was teaching at Johns Hopkins in the Sixties. I don't know, maybe hindsight is 20-20, but I always had a sixth sense about them. Something flaky about them I didn't trust. A vivid memory: whenever I came home from college on vacation the Kayes would say, "We must have you over before you go back to school." But then they wouldn't call. It happened once, twice, a dozen times. I became embarrassed for them every time they said it. They didn't notice.

Dr. Kaye was the first personal friend David told about the illness, after Mom. He told him in confidence. Explained he wasn't ready to tell the whole world. Dad cried, I'm sure. Not because he told me he had, but because he cried almost every time he said it out loud. He was telling Kaye, he said, because he and Pauli needed support and wanted the Kayes—their close friends—to understand what they were going through.

But soon after that conversation, the Kayes dropped out of sight. And that's when David decided to say something. He called Kaye to his office, told him he didn't feel they were being supportive. "Supportive?! What's that? What the hell does supportive mean?" Ted Kaye screamed. He was on the defensive. "We're friends of yours, we're here. Just call on us when you need us," he said, slamming the door behind him as he left Dad's office.

Supportive. It's become a big word in our family. A theme word. Attitude more than action. General more than specifics. It's the kind of thing; if you don't know what it is, no one can really tell you.

After that confrontation, Sally, Ted's wife, started calling. Every night, around seven. "How are you? How's David? Pretty much the same, huh. Well, that's good. I'll talk to you again tomorrow." The calls were a chore, routine; every night after dinner and before washing the dishes, something to check off her list. After a few weeks I guess she decided it was as silly as we thought and stopped.

The current update on the Kayes: We see them every six or eight weeks. It's hard to make arrangements with them: they seem to have a million and one things on their schedule. When they finally locate a free block of time for us, something "catastrophic" —a fender-bender, the appearance of a horrid guest from out of town—inevitably occurs. When they appear, they come in with a big whoosh and a hullabaloo, looking disheveled, wearing large floppy hats and toting big brown shopping bags. They sit down, have a few laughs and share old times. Then off they go, like cats on a hot tin roof, can't sit still. Life is hectic and time is money.

October 1, 1981

We've retreated into the warmth of an old, time-and-distance-tested womb of friendships. People like Godfrey and Lorraine Getz (the former Lorraine Cohen from medical school), who now also live in the United States, in Chicago. Over the years, double dates turned into family get-togethers, political rallies into quiet evenings of debate and discussion. Time and distance have not dulled the bonds. When Michael was attending the University of Chicago, the Getz family made their household his home away from home. My parents love these gentle, intelligent people. Dad calls Godfrey "a prince." And when the two of them are together, there is something noble and transcendant, a majestic quality, to the way those two discuss science, literature, the world.

We also rely more and more on our old friends from Baltimore, people like Patsy and Tony Perlman, Howard and Jane Cohen, Barbara Koeppel, and Eddie Berman. There are no doubts here; we know they will be with us. Some of those friendships were forged during a crisis, back in Baltimore in 1962.

We don't talk about Lisa very much. It's still painful, something we prefer to keep submerged. Lisa was born two years after I was. From the beginning my parents knew something was wrong. She had blotchy skin and a milky film over her eyes. They took her to see Tony Perlman, our pediatrician, and he recommended Dr. Walsh, a well-known ophthalmologist. In Walsh's offices their worst suspicions were confirmed: Lisa had a fatal neurological illness, and she probably wouldn't live for more than a year. But that wasn't the worst of it: tuberous sclerosis is familial, and it was highly likely that Michael or I would be affected. And they certainly shouldn't risk having any more children.

My parents were devastated. But then one of the young residents asked to take a look at Lisa. He remembered reading about a disease similar to tuberous sclerosis—essentially the same symptoms, but very rare, and without a trace of a genetic component. The resident did a thorough examination, and then went back to the literature to locate the article. He reviewed the case with Dr. Walsh, and together they examined the baby. Walsh was relieved to find he had made a mistake. The resident was right; the disease was not hereditary.

Until then, Tony had been little more than the family doctor. But he stood by my parents through all of this. He visited every evening while Lisa was struggling. Little could be done to alleviate her pain, and she died when she was only five months old. After she died Tony invited the family up to Maine for the summer. He knew we didn't have relatives in the United States, and he knew we didn't have much money, but he thought my parents deserved a vacation. He and Patsy had three children—

two boys a few years older than Michael, and a daughter my age, Ellen—and he was sure we'd get along. "C'mon," he said, "we've got a huge summer cottage up there, right on the lake. It's beautiful. There's tons of room and it won't cost you a penny."

At first Mom and Dad were reluctant, not wanting to be the "poor relations." But Tony made it difficult to say no. He called every few days to see if they had changed their mind, and finally my parents caved in. It turned out to be a wonderful week and the beginning of a long-lasting friendship. Morning dips in the lake, blueberry pancakes made with freshly picked blueberries, fishing, rowing, and canoeing. Patsy knew all the edible berries in the woods, the sound of the pileated woodpecker, and how to make pear jam. When the Perlmans' dog got chewed up in a fight, Tony and David sewed him back together with what they remembered from their surgery rotations in school.

The Perlmans visited us in Israel, and later, when we returned to the United States, an annual Thanksgiving reunion became a tradition for our two families. So, six months after the diagnosis, Tony and Patsy had flown down. Tony knew something was wrong right away. He had also trained at Witwatersrand, and had that keen Wits eye. "Great clinical intuition," Dad always said. And it was true. The moment he stepped off the plane, Tony knew. He took one look at David's walking and said, "Sure you don't have some degeneration of the anterior horn cell, Dov?" but David brushed him off, "Nah." He wanted them to have a good holiday weekend together. He could call Tony later; it would be easier over the phone.

But Dad dreaded making that phone call. Luckily he didn't have to. Because Tony called us. He called as soon as he and Patsy had arrived back in Baltimore. And Pauline told him.

After that, the Perlmans started visiting more frequently, in spite of the expense and time involved in flying down from Baltimore. They were grieving, but they never let us see it. Instead they came down, suitcases jam-packed with "real" bagels from the famous Baltimore delis, salmon caught and smoked by Tony himself, honey from the beehives they kept on their farm. They were doers. If they visited in the winter they shoveled snow for us; in the spring they checked for termites. Most importantly, they filled the house with a feeling . . . like relatives, like family.

Not long after Pauline told the Perlmans what the limp meant, David realized he had to tell our other Yankee friends. Mom and Dad had made plans to meet with the Cohens for a weekend of opera in New York that winter, but David knew he couldn't make it. They had to cancel, but David kept putting off the painful phone call. Finally there was no way around it. So one Sunday afternoon, when Dana and Leora were safely out of the way (this was in the winter of 79–80, when the kids still didn't know), he and Pauline sat down to call.

Howard answered the phone. "Well, it's time we heard from you. Ready for the big *Madama Butterfly?*" he asked.

"Actually, that's what we're calling about, Howard," David said. "I've been having some trouble getting around. I mentioned it to you a couple of months ago."

"Yes, I know. But you're still swimming and taking care of yourself, aren't you?"

"Well, yes, but—but, my mobility has been severely curtailed. I just don't think we'll be able to make the New York trip. It's too much for me."

"But David. Listen. I'll drive my car up and meet you at the airport. We'll reserve a wheelchair for the Picasso exhibit. And I'll be there, I'll help you. Hell, I'll carry you—"

"No, you don't understand, Howard. Howard, I've got a serious illness. I've got ALS."

As Dad said it, his voice cracked. He handed the receiver over to Pauline and broke down crying. Those three words broke him every time. I have ALS. Not you or he or she. Me. I have it. I can't disown it. I can't take it out and throw it away. I have it. I'm stuck with it.

Mom took the phone and told Howard she would call back later. Dad was bawling like a child. But they pulled themselves together —Dana and Leora were due home shortly.

A few days later a letter arrived.

Dear David and Pauline,

You are very often in our thoughts and now constantly so since we spoke to you on Sunday. The problem you face is our problem too, because you occupy a large space in our lives, and we perhaps in yours. It is difficult and usually unnecessary to verbalize expressions of friendship and love—especially in our relationship with you—but urgent in time of crisis, because that is when all one's resources must be mustered up. You must consider us one of your resources.

We feel so strongly about this because you are among the handful of people in the world whom we look up to. It would be boring for you to read a long listing of the qualities that we admire and try to emulate in you both. But surely part of that inventory is a fierce determination to meet adversity. It is not in you to give up, and we know you will not do so now. We realize how easily we say this, understanding that the doing is yours. We want to come and see you soon, to encourage you, to help in any way we can. A steady stream of visitors will not be welcome, so let us know a good time. We feel ever more close to you and wish we could literally reach out and touch you.

You may consider this a love letter from,

Howard and Jane

October 3

It's been wild around here for the past two weeks. The phone hasn't stopped ringing since the *New England Journal of Medicine* published Dad's article about the first round of experiments on the male contraceptive. The story got picked up by UPI and next thing we knew it was on the front page of the *Washington Post* and in the *New York Times,* and Cable News was knocking at the door. *Omni* magazine is doing a feature story and a hundred radio stations from all over have called—including one from Australia. Poor Dad, he'd like to grant interviews to all of them—and he explains it so well, in layman's language—but his voice tires out. I have to screen the calls, torn between "famous Daddy" and "tired Dad, not to be strained."

The good news of the study is that the contraceptive Dad developed managed to reduce sperm production by seventy-five to one hundred percent, also reducing sperm motility. The bad news is that some of the men became impotent after six weeks on the drug, even though they all returned to normal after being taken off it.

It's interesting: the first question women reporters always ask is: "How will women be able to trust men to take it?" The first question the male reporters invariably ask is: "What about the *impotence*?"

The next step in the research will be, naturally, to try and solve that very problem by giving supplements of testosterone. It's a long process; the results will take another year to come in. But Dad got another grant of $350,000 over the next three years. The grant reviews were highly complimentary! One of the few times I've seen David show off. "Take a look at this—they couldn't find anything wrong with the application. And let me tell you, it wasn't 'cause they weren't trying."

Some of the comments:

"The proposal is a carefully prepared clinical project and designed with excellent experimental efficiency. . . ."

"This work is excellent and the present application which addresses important problems that need answers anticipates the same high quality . . ."

"This proposal will provide important information on these points with a high degree of probability because protocols are presented to examine in detail effects of LHRH on the testes and the pituitary with excellent efficiency of experimental design. The attention of the investigator to other actions of LHRH on the testes is laudable and illustrates the competence of this laboratory to study these problems . . ."

A few days later

Page proofs of Dad's endocrinology text have arrived from the publisher. He's busy proofreading, examining diagrams, figures, and photos. Dad is glad to be busy.

Dad pretends.

Today he had a phone call from an old friend in Canada. "How are you getting along?" the friend asked. "Oh, I'm just having some problems with my legs," David answered. "I'm just having some problems getting around."

Even to his own siblings he pretended. After he returned from South Africa, Mom told him he had to write and tell his relatives the truth. The letter he wrote was full of medical terms, statistics, and obscure references. Towards the end, one sentence in particular stood out: "This condition has a high incidence of mortality."

"It was a bunch of gobbledygook," Mom said. "You had to be a fortune-teller to know what it meant."

Maybe this is why people respond the way they do. Perhaps they think David is covering up, expecting them to play along—and they can't bring themselves to do so. He never mentions his illness, either directly or in passing. Maybe they think he's trying to get a message across: I'm okay, you're okay. This thing that's happening to me is no concern of yours. Or maybe they interpret it as pride: I can handle this. You're not needed.

Our family has become closer. At the end of the day we gather in the den, a small room with big windows, a warm shag rug, and comfortable sofa. It's our center and we convene there, watch the evening news and drink hot tea, open the mail and talk about "it." The den is our headquarters. There we discuss our options and plan strategy. It's us against the world.

Yesterday Mom brought up what I was thinking about just a few days earlier. She talked slowly, it was difficult for her. But, she said, she couldn't help wondering. Perhaps their friends were put off by their reluctance to discuss the illness. Perhaps they feel David is being secretive and trying to shut them out.

"Well, in one aspect you're right," David said. "I don't like talking about the illness, and I'm not about to start talking about it. It's very painful for me. I've never been the sort to spill my troubles out, it's not the nature of my personality, whether they are personal problems or work problems. I don't dwell on them, I never have. I've always been an activist. That is the way I cope. I'm not going to change just because some people disapprove of the way I'm handling this. This is the way that I cope. I would not be able to function—and enjoy my life—if I did it any other way. I think a real friend will accept what's easiest and most comfortable for me."

"Well, Dovi, then I'm not sure you can complain if people get the wrong message," Pauli said.

"No, you see, I disagree with you. I absolutely cannot accept that," David said. "I don't put people off. On the contrary. I greet people even when they don't greet me. I go out of my way to make conversation with my colleagues and put them at ease, even when I should be concentrating on every step so I don't fall. So I disagree with that. I think the message I send out is clear. 'I want to be your friend. I'm ill, and I don't like talking about my disability. But I am reaching out for your friendship and I hope you can respect my wishes.' If people are put off by that, and won't have a relationship except under circumstances prescribed by them—when I'm the one who's sick—then okay. But handling the illness this way is what's comfortable for me."

"Anyway, Mom, I think that's just an excuse when people say that," Leora said. "I mean, if you went and told them everything and cried your heart out to them, they wouldn't like that either. Then they'd say you're handling it really badly, wearing your heart on your sleeve and stuff."

"Well, I guess I'm like Daddy. I've never done that and it's just not in my personality to do that," Pauline said. But it was true that people used it as an excuse. Someone told our next-door neighbor: "She's a very private person. I don't like to ask, I wouldn't want to intrude."

"It's kind of a no-win situation. People will find any excuse if they really don't want to deal with it," Dana said.

It's true. A Catch-22. I remember seeing Mrs. Kaye in the bookstore. She heard Dad wasn't going to work anymore, she said, she supposed he was very bitter. No, I told her, he's very philosophical about it. He stays home and gets a lot of work done right in our living room, I said. She seemed disappointed. Well, I guess that's the only way he can get his mind off it—by burying himself in his work.

When I told David the story, he said, "That's true. But I think the message we send out is very clear. We have the concerts; we invite people over. I think our message is unambiguous."

David was so lively, so strong. Talking to him you could forget. He'd be telling you about his work on the male contraceptive and his eyes would light up. Sitting in his big armchair with his eyes riveted on you. "Our volunteers have been wonderful. It never would have come this far without their cooperation and dedication . . ." You'd be listening to him speak and you'd be carried away. He was so enthusiastic, and he had so much invested in his fight—in life—it seemed impossible he could fail. And you forgot the walking cane leaning against the chair, forgot he would need your help to get up.

Maybe that was what bothered people: the forgetting, and then the jolt. The shock. Each time, all over again. Death creeping up, even on the seemingly invincible. Even on the enthusiastic, the young, the best, the brightest, the fighters. Out of nowhere, and for no reason. It made you feel terribly defenseless, vulnerable and unprepared.

"I can't believe what's happening to us; I can't believe what we've become." Mom.

And me too. I'm very self-conscious about the fact that I stay home and nurse my father. I hate telling people, and when I'm introduced I dread the "And what do you do?" I long for chitchat about office developments, the stuff of silly daily routine. Someone asked me out for lunch and when I said I couldn't go out during the day he said, "What is this, a Victorian novel?" I do feel like a character in a novel. I know her well. She is described as plain and is quiet, subdued. She wears dresses ten years out of style; the house is dim and when her father dies she marries the wrong person, a man much older than herself and very mean. I'm convinced that people can tell just by looking at me. There's a distinguishing mark, a sign on my forehead: DYING FATHER. And that's me: girl with dying father. Set apart. People look at me with orphan's eyes, sick dog looks. I can hear them, I know what they say. "Oh, you know her father has that horrible illness. . . ." "Really? How awful. Poor girl." Me. Poor girl. I was never poor girl before. I was talented girl, sweet girl, rebellious girl, horrible girl. Never poor girl.

I hate meeting new people; I hate explaining the situation anew, and I'm convinced it'll scare them off. Who'd want to get involved with such a messy situation? And what a demand to start off with, as a friend in need. So I wheedle my way through conversations, learning how to avoid the truth without lying. Yes, I'm just finishing up some courses, living at home, trying to save money.

I'm a princess, an heiress, a gypsy. . . . I read a lot. . . . I am ashamed that I don't work, that at twenty-one I still live at home, and I feel that somehow being me is wrong, that if I were someone else I wouldn't be caught dead in this situation, my father wouldn't be sick. No matter how much I intellectualize it ("It hits one in one hundred thousand; that one just happened to be Dad"), I still think somehow it was our fault that fate singled us out ("Well, then why our house, why not across the street, down the road?"). And it is such a horrible illness, a freak illness, a shameful illness; dark and evil and monstrous and inexplicable. Many ALS patients think their disease was sent directly, a curse from God.

In spite of all my logical protestations, here it is: I have accepted the bad luck looks, the orphan eyes, the guilt of the victim. There are other things too, things I can share with Dad and he can advise me about. I've changed, and I don't like this change. Very settled. Creature comforts. Bourgeois. No desire to volunteer at the shelter, or print a radical newspaper. I want a home, sunshine on the kitchen table, healthy children. I swore I'd never say, "I used to be young and idealistic." But I don't trust in action, I don't believe anything can change, and I don't have the energy, besides.

Dad says I'm going through a phase. It's natural I should be preoccupied with self and home now. It'd almost be unnatural if I weren't. I don't have any excess emotional energy for causes. I'm preserving my resources, and it makes sense. It's a temporary survival tactic.

But I'm very fatalistic. Everything seems predetermined. Here Dad didn't smoke or drink all his life, and he got ALS. Then there's a guy who smoked nonfilter cigarettes and drank corn whiskey who climbed mountains until he was eighty-three and died in his sleep, sweet dreams.

October 30
Dad couldn't walk today. He kept falling back into Willis' arms. He couldn't get it together. Legs like overboiled noodles. We had to carry him the last two feet to the chair. He has no muscle; he walks on balance.

We didn't tell Mom. She gets so anxious at each new deterioration, as if it weren't inevitable. "But you promised me you were going to get better!" she pouts at him.

Later on he said, "I feel like a twit today."

"Well, you are a bit of a twit," she said. "But why, did something happen today?" She knows him so well.

"No," he white-lies, "I just feel like a twit."

"Well, you're a twit for feeling like a twit," Mom said. "How's that?" And then she was crouching over his chair and hugging him, "Oh, Dovi, don't feel like a twit, man. . . ."

November 10, 1981

Though I had talked to Dad about the bourgeois thing, I never could bring myself to talk about my self-image. He knew something was wrong, but every time he reached, I ran. I couldn't tell him because he would blame himself, and anyway, what could he do about it? Maybe it'll help to talk, he kept saying; it helps to talk things over. But it was easier to run. He wouldn't let me off the hook, and finally I told him. I told him I felt like a bum, useless. "That's crazy," he said. "What you're doing is valuable; you're doing a wonderful thing staying with me . . . don't deprecate it. It's hard work; it requires patience and courage and maturity. It just so happens that you're in a convenient position to do it—Michael and Dana and Leora are in school, and Mom has to work. But if you weren't here we'd have to pay someone a fortune to come in, and it'd be a drain on our resources. That doesn't make what you're doing any less valuable. You can't go on doing it forever—you have to go back to graduate school and make a career for yourself. I hope you're thinking about that. . . .

"And you're wrong—it's not something anyone could do. Trained nurses get paid to do this sort of thing, and naturally it's much nicer for me that it's you. Ten years from now you'll look back and you won't have any regrets, because you were here when you were able to, you had a chance to help and you did, and you stuck it out . . . so don't say you're a bum just because you're not earning a wage. You're not a bum. Not one scintilla of you is a bum. You're thoughtful and sensitive and kind, and you're doing a valuable job. You've matured so much in the past year, and you're a wonderful companion to me."

Dad says all this in his deep, slow voice. I hold his hands, which are shaking and flickering underneath my fingers. My first impulse is to let go but I hold fast.

"You have to rely on your own resources. It has to come from within. You can't be bitter—be optimistic about the future. You'll make it. It'll be hard and it might take a lot of effort, but you'll make it. And you have to support each other, the five of you."

We talk a lot now, Dad and I. I still feel that resistance within myself, that drive to stick to your guns, not give in, keep a straight face. I feel terrible for burdening him with my hang-ups and petty neuroses when he's so sick. "Don't," he says, "you do so much for me, let me help you too. And I'm not going to be here much longer. You've got to talk these things out and maybe I can help; I'm a little bit older, a little bit wiser."

As we talk, new issues emerge, fears I'm not totally aware of—my future, my career, getting back on the track, how to make a living from my writing. For me it's just a haze, but he talks concretely: journalism, grad school, Master's programs, GRE's.

Sometimes Mom says to him, "I don't want you to go!" Like a spoiled child. "I'm not too keen on it myself," he says, making light. Then we girls have a spat, a miscommunication and he says, "You're babies, I can't leave you. Don't clam up—talk about it. Talking is to resolve." And when Mom is down on herself he talks to me about self-esteem. "You've got to have self-esteem. In a way that's all you've got. If your mother thought she was worth ten percent of what she's really worth, she'd be in great shape."

You have to be careful. Self-esteem is a trick done with mirrors. If you keep your eyes fixed on the image you think you see in the glass, it will control you. It will have you mimic it instead of following your movements. You become its shadow; it comes to own you. Like the sane man placed behind grilles in a mental institution, you begin acting the part. Seeing someone who has avoided me in the past I shrivel up like a silhouette to avoid the embarrassment of an encounter. Later I will be furious, having allowed the behavior, giving my tacit approval by shrinking, making myself small and scarce. The only way out is to force yourself to look away, smash the glass, cause a confrontation.

* * *

Michael was here this weekend. Dad cried when he walked into the room the day he arrived. Then as he was leaving on Sunday evening Dad told him the visit had been very good for his morale. "This visit has been very uplifting for me. I've been very well emotionally for the past three days and I'll look forward to your next visit. Now work like a dog and hang in there!"

"You too," Michael said, meaning it.

"Don't worry," Dad said, "I have every intention of doing just that."

He doesn't talk about himself much, old Dad, but yesterday he told me that in his dreams, as in Dana's, he is always mobile and doing something active—swimming long, long strokes, running the dogs, just walking.

November 18

People again. Apparently some woman told another friend of my mother's that she would very much like to visit David but that "I hear Pauline discourages visitors." Great excuse. The fact of the matter is that the woman is scared to death and hasn't been near any of us in months. Needless to say, Dana, Leora, and I were infuriated. We wondered who the little birdie was—a drop-out rationalizing, no doubt. But Mom took it like old hat. "She'd prefer if I did discourage visitors," she said. "That would be a lot easier for her than making a short visit."

Other things get Mom down though. Personal encounters. She went to the supermarket and rolled her cart by two women who haven't called or come over for two years. Apparently they were more embarrassed than she. Still, the way they slink away, as if you're not a real person to them anymore. As if you had raped or hatchet-slaughtered. As if you were an untouchable, Bigfoot. The elephant man.

And it seems we should be spared the hassles, these daily nuisances, the battery of the car dying because you left the lights on, the triple A putting you on hold and forgetting about you, stuff like that. But Dad always laughs. "Gosh, I've gone all day without watching TV!" Well, that proves it's not physically addictive."

A few days later:

I'm real proud of Mom. We went to the opening of a local book fair last night. She almost copped out because she knew that the Meyersons would be there, and that Sherrie would run up and gush all over her. Gush, gushing, gushes, gushed. You feel awful saying, hey, cut the crap. But if "they're not worth getting upset about," then what do you make of the years of conversations, shared jokes, evenings spent together, warmth you were sure of? My parents really liked the Meyersons—they're interesting, open, lively. About six months ago Dad had called to invite them over for dinner. But Mr. Meyerson's "no" was too quick, it sounded like he had decided ahead of time, didn't even need to consult his calendar. "Well, say something to her," I told Mom. "Don't let her get away with it. I'll protect you."

So who do we run into in the first booth? The Meyersons. And just like Mom predicted, Sherrie comes up, hugs, kisses, "How are you?" the whole spiel.

"Actually, we've been very disappointed in you," Mom said. "We haven't heard from you in ages, and you know David's been so ill."

"Oh, I was so busy this summer, we were all busy, running around, just didn't have any free—"

"You make time when it's important," Mom insisted, quietly.

"Pauline, we think about you all the time. Don't we, honey?" Sherrie said, and turned to her husband for reassurance, then back to Mom. "We're always talking about you. Always. The children always ask about you. And we're always trying to find out how you are—"

"That doesn't help us though—listen, I don't want to make a scene. I just wanted to let you know how we feel. We felt very close to you, when we had good luck . . . Now we're having bad luck—"

"C'mon, Sher," Mr. Meyerson interrupted. "She's right. Let's not make a scene. C'mon, let's go."

"No." Sherrie said, "Pauline, this is crazy. I love you. I really love you. What can I do?"

"Just call us."

"But why don't you call me? Our house is so difficult, David can't get there and I can't just invite myself over—"

"Of course you can. Why not?"

"I can?" Sherrie turned to her husband. "You see? Oh, I hate it, I hate it! But, Pauline, really. You don't know how difficult it is to be with someone who's ill. . . ."

"Oh, come on now. . . ." Pauline said, shaking her head. Hell, if anyone knows . . .

"Pauline, I'll call you. I'll call you and we'll come by. Send David my love."

"I will."

"Pauline?"

"Yes?"

"It'll be difficult the first time."

Next day:

I really didn't think we'd see the Meyersons again—I thought it would be too difficult for all involved. But they called and are coming for coffee tonight. I think it was a genuine misunderstanding. Glad we got it resolved.

Mom is getting gutsy. Said to one of her colleagues, in her department, "You know, it's incredible. Neither you nor any of the other senior members of the staff ever acknowledge David's illness. You're completely unsupportive. You never ask me how he is or how we're managing. You keep the conversation strictly on work and never let it stray from work-related issues."

The colleague had nothing to say to this. "Remember that time you came over to drop off that book?" Pauline asked, and she nodded. "David was walking down the driveway with his walker and you didn't say hello to him. Why? I just want to understand. Here's a sick man; why didn't you greet him? It's not as if you don't know him."

"He looked agonized," the colleague answered.

"All the more reason to greet him, don't you think?" Mom answered.

"I hate it when people don't ask, but on the other hand, when they ask a thousand questions—'Can he still eat? Can he swallow? Can he breathe all right? Can he chew? Can he feed himself?'—

I go crazy, I swear," I said. "It may sound like nothing they do is ever any good but . . ."

"But that's not true," Dad said. "There are many people who are comfortable and make us feel comfortable. Most people are sensitive and don't ask all those things. 'How is he?' is hard enough to handle, and they know that."

"But what do you do when they don't ask—when you know they know? When there's no question that they know David is sick and they avoid any topic that might lead to it? You feel like you're helping in a cover-up, like you're an accomplice in their avoidance and insensitivity. What can you do?"

"Just say something like, 'I'm surprised you don't ask about my father. You know he's been so ill.' That can be said very benignly, but it gets the point across."

"What I can't stand is when I run into people and they say, 'We're thinking of you.' 'We think about you all the time.' I don't believe it," Pauline said. "They're not thinking about us all the time—I'm not thinking about them, that's for sure. That's just to make them feel less guilty."

"Sometimes they say—or write—'We're praying for you,'" Dad said. "That's okay, I accept that. They believe, and that's their way of helping. . . ."

"See, though?" I said. "I'm just the opposite. I can't stand that!"

"But why?"

"I find it offensive. It offends me. Implicit in it is a kind of assumption that someone is up there taking charge of all this, in control of this. Of this, right here. So the reason you're sick is because you did something wrong, and maybe if they say enough Hail Mary's God will forgive you even though you are a nonbeliever. In a sneaky kind of self-righteous way it implies that the reason they're well is because they pray."

"I understand what she's saying," Dad said. "It just goes to show you that everyone's different. It doesn't bother me. They want to pray—let them pray. Doesn't bother me."

"I'll tell you. I had a friend who was constantly talking about how God will take care of everything. Just in general. And I said, 'Well, where is your God? Why isn't He taking care of my father?'

And she said, 'Maybe He is.' I didn't say anything but I was thinking, 'Helluva way to take care of him, huh?' I hate that 'mysterious ways' stuff. The whole idea that good comes out of bad. Even if it does, it doesn't cancel out the bad, it's just in addition. The loss is still there. Even if there is an afterlife, you're still lost to me. I can see some good that's come from this illness, sure. We've grown closer as a family, maybe. But we did that, not God. I refuse to attribute that to Him or Her or anyone. I think we deserve the credit for that. Hell, a lot of families go to the dogs when this happens. The spouse will just split, and the kids will go bonkers. And let's say, just for the sake of argument, that God did do it. God thinks a close family is a valuable thing, so valuable it's worth it. Then why break it up with a death? The basic theological refutation seems to be that everything bad that humans do is their fault, but everything good we do 'He' gets credit for. God gets to have His cake and eat it too."

Dad always ends these discussions with a pep talk.

"I just hope you won't be bitter," he says "It'll scar you for the rest of your lives if you are. All these hurts would be trivial if I weren't sick, and no one made me sick—not even the Kayes, nobody. If you are going to be bitter then there's no reason for me to struggle to stay alive; it defeats the purpose. So try to use this as a learning experience, and grow from it instead of shrinking and retreating from the world."

"Twenty-one is too young to give up on people," he says to me. "Seventy-one is too young! You and Mom are alike; you both give a lot so you expect a lot. I expect very little from people. It's a question of whether the glass is half full or half empty. I've been surprised by how many people have stood by us, have pulled through. You have to be careful and judge before being too intimate and vulnerable. Don't give too quickly; don't give up too quickly."

My father is such an optimist that when I walk him to his room and say, "Boy, it's cold in here, isn't it?" he says, "No, it's just the change in temperature."

When he talks he fills me with hope. I think of Elaine Fleming, who brings over enormous jugs of chicken soup for him, even though she knows all the chicken soup in the world can't make him better, but she wants to do something, and what can she do? Or Mr. Miller, our handyman, who came to tinker with the heating. He couldn't locate the problem but seemed to have gotten the furnace going anyway. "Well, like they say in the army," he said, "when you can't do anything more, just salute." Then he whispered to me in a low voice gruff from too many cigarettes, "How's my friend doin'? How's my friend? He gettin' better or gettin' worse, how's he doin'? Wish you could tell me he's getting better—if you can you call me up right away, hear?"

Every week there are packages from South Africa. Chocolate bars, fig jam, custard powder, anchovy paste, long-sleeved shirts, winter pajamas, rose tea.

And lot of letters. From patients. "Dear Dr. Rabin, I will always be grateful for the help that you gave me. I am now 5'9" and weigh 175 pounds. Still working on that mustache. . . ."

And their families. "I appreciate your interest in my mother and your taking time out of your busy schedule to help her. Thank you for taking the time to care. That's what makes you the beautiful person everyone loves."

And old colleagues from Hopkins: "I have just learned of the extent of your illness. I can't tell you how concerned I am about your health and wanted to pass on my best wishes for the difficult time I know you must be going through. I think of you frequently and wanted to let you know what a profound influence you have had on my life. The days at Hopkins were filled with great excitement and you provided guidance, stimulus, and innovative thought that made that period so productive. . . ."

"It is a pleasure to remember the middle 1960's when I worked for you. . . . That certainly was an active and productive period. Your kindness and thoughtfulness made it possible for me to work and be a mother to my children at the same time. I have been very fortunate to work with people like you, people I admire and respect. You were very generous and patient in sharing your knowledge. I am indebted to you for the start you gave my career. My best wishes to you and your family. May God keep you in His care."

We have a whole drawer full of letters, photos of Dad, articles about the contraceptive research. One letter is from a lab technician at Hadassah, saying they've moved to a new lab and had hoped David would be returning.

The new boss sits on his ivory chair and doesn't interest himself in the lab, much less in the people. We're not used to that kind of attitude; you spoiled us.

Winter is taking its time getting here. The weather is wonderful, blue skies and pleasant sunshine, at least there's that to be proud of. On the other hand the economic and political spheres are not flourishing. Prices are going up, salaries are going down, and the fights between the parties get more and more vicious every day. The holidays have passed and no miracles have taken place, and this country needs a big miracle to get it back on the tracks.

David, we think of you often, and we always miss you. It's a pity you aren't here. The energy and love of life that you gave us and the lab are not here now. The atmosphere is completely different, impersonal and formal, and even though it's been several years since you left, it's hard to become accustomed to it. So David, it's a pity that you're so far away, but still, we remember you and think only good of you.

David has no regrets about leaving Israel. If at times he regrets that we didn't leave sooner, other times he is proud that we stuck it out for as long as we did. It was a difficult decision but we made it. We re-established ourselves in this country—we didn't become drifters or hobos; we got on with our lives. The Israel years were the most critical and the most traumatic, but Dad's hunch, he says, is they had nothing to do with the illness. Regrets? Well, you can always find place for them if you want to.

Mom says there's no evidence of psychosomatic factors in ALS. One out of one hundred thousand people are struck every year. That's chance, fate, luck. There are some things you can control: how many cigarettes you smoke, whether you get enough exercise, whether you appreciate each day. Other things intrude; they drop out of the sky. That's a crucial factor that holistic health theories à la Norm Cousins don't take into account: You can be responsible for your health; you can't be responsible for your illness.

My gut feeling is simply: if Dad couldn't get better, who could? Florence Ruderman, in a scathing review of Norman Cousins' book *Anatomy of an Illness* (*Commentary*, May 1980), says of "those who think that the operation of their body's natural processes is somehow due to their own brilliance or originality" that "this is the mentality of the cock who perceives clearly that his crowing made the sun rise." Although many doctors hailed the book, she said that members of the medical profession want to believe that patients can wish themselves well if they believe it strongly enough: "Consciously or unconsciously, many doctors react to the incurably ill with hostility. Doctors, too, want miracles. Doctors, too, want a guru . . . to absolve the profession from failures and blunders." So although it may be said that you cannot get better if you don't want to, it doesn't follow that you can get better if *only* you want to.

But a much more important issue is involved. Holistic health theories, while offering hope, are implicitly dangerous. "If you don't get better, it's your fault," they say. Like a modern secular form of the old religious dictum, "You're punished for being bad and rewarded for being good," such theories guarantee for the healthy the illusion that the world is safe and orderly, not haphazard and unpredictable. It also gives them a hip excuse to place the guilt on the victim and vindicate themselves—"You're handling the illness the wrong way." By casting aspersions on the illness—after all, the illness could have been averted—these theories belittle the very real anguish and pain that the patient and family are suffering, and reinforce their guilt and negative self-esteem, which have already been compounded by the avoidance and evasive behaviors of friends and colleagues.

Susan Sontag has explained in *Illness as Metaphor* that the imagery and alleged causes attached to mysterious illnesses grow out of the fears and obsessions of the current age. In the twentieth century we had the sexual revolution and it was acceptable to express feelings; the "cancer personality" therefore is one who represses his or her feelings. In the nineteenth century, when it wasn't acceptable to express emotion, tuberculosis was blamed on an excess of feeling. But the cause of tuberculosis, we now know, was not a personality type or a psychological response or anything of the sort. It was a bacillus. A bacterium.

December 10, 1981

Further deterioration, just in the past week or so. Dad has lost some small movements: the ninety-degree turn from a forward stance to a sideways one; the ability to bring the fork all the way to his mouth. We've started a new morning routine, eliminating the one o'clock bathroom run. By being careful with liquids Dad can make it through the day until Mom comes home from work and can empty his bladder into a urinal in the living room or the den.

He has decided not to go out anymore. He says he's so tired by the time he gets wherever he's going that he can't enjoy it, and then there's still the return trip to worry about. All of us have tried to talk him out of this decision, but he is pretty hardheaded. He says everything he needs and wants is here; the people he loves are here, and his friends and colleagues come to him. A conversation of one hour's length tires him. "All I would prove by going to the hospital is that I can get there. That's machismo, ineffectual heroics. I'd rather stay at home and get some work done." Of course, we don't push it—he has so little control over his life; let him at least have control over such decisions.

He still laughs. We were walking to the living room, and I brushed against the wall accidentally, toppling down a print. It fell to the floor with a crash and Dad laughed. "Oooh! For a minute I thought that was me!"

I've been having strange aches and pains lately. My farsighted vision seems to be deteriorating. Itches and scratches and cramps. Fleas in the house? I've changed the linen, boiled my clothes, beat the mattresses, banished the dogs. The back of my thigh twitches and I turn around to catch it in the act, but it's quiet. Then a thread of my shoulder muscle moves. Again I turn around: too late. A jug of milk slips from my hands and I remember: slipping and tripping can be the first warning signs. And I'm so scared of having unhealthy children: cerebral palsy, leukemia, blindness, mental retardation. I can be healthy today but what about ten years from now? Five years? Tomorrow?

Mom and I synchronize our moods so they don't coincide. One on, one off; one up, one down. When she's upset I make myself hard and flat. I make myself concrete and practical. "I don't want him to die, even though he's suffering so much. There'll be such an emptiness when he's gone," she says. But he is going to die, I say. You have to know that. And then he'll be gone, and then he'll never be here again. I'm calm. I'm calm as long as I'm talking; then I go upstairs and close the door.

At night I lie down, feeling my breasts for lumps that are like hard grapes and don't move. Mom tells me she read in a medical journal—in several, in fact—if you have kids when you're young you decrease the chance of getting breast cancer. With the palm of my hand I go round and round breathing deeply. The knots in my stomach are ulcers; there are cancers in my ankles and under my kneecaps.

And before we go out David tells us to watch out, to be cautious, to drive slowly. "I can take anything," he says, "anything. But not if something happens to one of you kids."

Today Mom says she's going on strike. She can't stand going to work; she makes people there uncomfortable; she isn't wanted. She walks through the halls like a leper, like a person in a plastic bubble. The junior faculty were wonderful, and so were the students. But for some reason her peers . . . If someone would just encourage her, tell her they admire her continuing to work, tell her they think she's brave or strong. "How is David? How are you? How are you coping?" But no. The best they seem able to do is say, "Pauline, you look awful. You look really tired."

The next time someone tells her she looks tired, she's going to scream, she says.

On second thought, the next time someone tells her she looks tired, she's going to say: "You don't look so hot yourself."

A few years ago a young medical student came to see her. The woman was going through a rough time—new in town, rough first year in school, having a hard time meeting people. Pauline helped her, encouraged her. When she finally settled down, graduated, and married, Mom sent her a gift. The thank-you note that followed thanked for more than the gift. "Your help to me was invaluable. I hope that if, at any time in the future, you

need help, I can be of encouragement and support as you were
to me." But ever since David's illness even the young doctor's
casual visits had ceased.—Why? If Pauline ever needed help,
surely this is the time?

A week later:

At Dad's insistence I went to see a doctor, a friend of his. Real
nice guy. When the nurse came in he said to her, "This is Dr.
Rabin's daughter. See any resemblance?"

"How about that?" she said, and gave me a big smile. "How's
our favorite doctor doing?"

I gave the doctor a list of symptoms. Then he left the room
while I undressed. Lying on the cot in the all-white room I had
a feeling of safeness and quiet, a curtain between me and the
world. I almost wanted to stay. But the doctor couldn't find
anything wrong with me. He did scrapes and searches and cul-
tures, but nothing. No lumps under my arms; no fleas or mites or
lice; no crabs or bites or bumps. He gave me some moisturizing
lotion—it could be dry skin, don't take too many hot baths. It
could be the latter stages of hepatitis, but that's absurd. And then,
it could be psychosomatic, but you better ask your mother
about that.

Then he asked me how Dad was, and whether ALS is hereditary. I told him, rarely. He started figuring out the statistical
probabilities and I turned away, stared at the wall. There was
a Hallmark poster with daisies on it that said, "Happiness is
making a bouquet out of the flowers you have on hand." I
concentrated on the lettering.

December 31

There's a new crisis every day. Dad has lost whatever muscles
are responsible for keeping him upright in a chair, and he slides
forward until his rear end is right on the edge. We are constantly
readjusting his position. It's hard to lift him and place him
further back on the chair; he's pretty heavy and we worry about
the strain on our backs. We try reducing it by teamwork, one on
each side grabbing under the arms; on your marks—get set—go.
Or we try the knee trick: you stand facing him, match your knees

up with his, take his hands, and, pulling his trunk forward with your arms, you press his knees into the chair so his bum goes backward.

Dad has started taking infusions of plasma twice a week. Possibly there is some as yet unidentified but crucial substance in the blood that ALS patients lack. It sounds a bit like plasmapheresis but those experiments weren't conducted with fresh plasma necessarily, and perhaps this elusive substance doesn't stick around for a long time outside of the body. In any case, Dad says he is feeling better and wants to continue the treatment. The idea was that of Goodman, a friend and colleague from Vanderbilt. He procures the plasma and Jeremy, a researcher who works with David on the male contraceptive, comes over and rigs up a home-style I.V. using an iron hanger and a curtain rod to hang it up.

Stan, Dad's old friend and colleague, was here from Philly and he showed us some prophylactic back exercises. We're all pretty worried about our backs, as is Dad, who tries to plan his day with as few moves as possible—"I don't want to leave you a legacy of bad backs."

The "pelvic tilt" exercise: Lie on the floor on your back and try to round out the spinal column so that it nestles against the floor instead of leaving that gap in the small of the back you can usually slip your hand under. You use your stomach muscles to do this, and you tilt your pelvis forward. Hence the name. Tilt and relax, tilt and relax, several times a day.

Swimming is also supposed to be effective as preventive therapy.

January 1982
I'm going through a new phase now—a new kind of anger. Everyone says it's okay, Dad even says it's normal ("Living with chronic illness is very difficult"), but it feels rotten. And it's him I'm angry with, angry at him for being so stubborn, for being so patient and understanding, for being so damn right all the time. Angry at him for giving orders while he just sits there; angry at him for just sitting there. And I think: my God, I have so little

time and I'm spending it being angry at him. Angry at him because I can't love him. Because every time I think of how much
I love him I feel the hot feeling in my face and change the subject.

"I get so angry at you sometimes—so angry!" I said, when I
went in to say good night.
"Why?" he said, ready and able to tackle the problem. "What
is it I do?"
"See? There you go again. You're so damn right all the time!"
"I hardly talk anymore though."
"You make me so mad sometimes!" I said, inarticulate and
embarrassed.
"But why? This is important."
"She's angry at the illness, Dovi," Mom said then. And suddenly
I realize: I protect myself with this anger; I protect the little girl
inside me who stamps her foot and says, "I want my Daddy!"
Every day I understand more about where the anger comes
from. I am angry at this frail, weak, and quiet man who has
replaced my cheerful, nimble father, joker and prankster. I
resent his attempts to imitate my father, with his quick smile and
his wit. You don't fool me, old man! I want my real father back.
Imposter! Take him away!

First snowfall

Goodman is terrific. I told him Dad really appreciated him
coming to help out with the plasma therapy, what with the snow
and all, and he said, "Hell, I'd come through a tornado to see
your Dad. He's a great guy, I enjoy talking to him." That was
good to hear. Dr. Kaye makes such a big deal out of his visits. He
hardly ever comes, though he keeps threatening he will. Once a
week he calls and makes excuses, tells me how busy he is, he'll
try to squeeze it in next week.

The Kayes are coming over this afternoon; there will be another
scene.
Later:
I was right. For a few minutes there I thought I was mistaken.
I could hear laughter and tall tales and I breathed a sigh of relief:

phew, it's all over. But then they rushed off mid-sentence after quick consultation with their watches. Sally had parted, giving Dad the perfunctory kiss on the cheek but not letting her eyes meet his. Mom said the whole visit seemed rehearsed: they had sat down, recited a repertoire of you-wouldn't-believe's and that-reminds-me's, and then left without even asking how David was getting along, without saying when they would be back.

"I don't get it. Didn't they grow up learning a friend in need is a friend indeed and all that?" Leora asked. "I thought everybody knew that stuff."

"Well, I think they did and that's why they feel obligated to come. I don't think they'd come otherwise. They obviously don't enjoy it," Mom said.

"I don't enjoy it. Their visits are agonizing to me. There's nothing genuine about them. Not a shred of sincerity," Dad said.

"It's really interesting, because we used to be a high priority item for them," Mike said. "When Dad was well—and we were important figures in the community—there was nothing they wouldn't do for us. But now we can't do anything for them any more. It's not as prestigious for them to be associated with us. Very interesting."

"I hate to admit it, but I think that may be true. My illness has made us less important in their eyes."

"Well, I don't understand why you continue to subject yourselves to their visits," I said.

"I know, Dov," Mom said. "They're not enjoyable to them; they're not enjoyable to us. What's the point? They're just begging to be relieved from the responsibility. Next time they call, why don't we say, 'Look, these visits aren't doing either of us any good so why don't we just discontinue them.' And end it there, quietly, without a fuss."

"Except they've got such big mouths," Dana said.

"People will be bound to ask them about us and they'll blame it on us and say we're bitter and angry and won't even see them— some of our closest friends—any more."

"And the worst thing about it is people will believe them because it's what they want to believe anyway," I said.

"Maybe that's a risk we have to take," Dana said. "I mean,

this is ridiculous. Every time they come here it's a major tragedy. And every time they leave we sit here and talk about it for hours."

"At some point we're going to have to weigh continuing these visits or letting go of them and living with the consequences," David said. "I agree with Dana. I think we have a right to protect ourselves. At some point we're going to have to put our foot down and do what's best for us."

It's an invisible tug of war.

Some interesting people stories:

I went out to lunch with a friend, and on the way she asked if I wouldn't mind stopping by Biff's house to see how he was doing, his father had just died. Suddenly? I asked. He'd had a heart condition, she explained, they were kind of expecting it but still. I don't know Biff well so I wasn't sure, but I said I didn't mind. So Biff joined us for lunch. Halfway through the meal my friend started bugging him—hey, we're going out partying tonight, right Biff? Two weeks ago, we made a date, you promised. Remember? C'mon. Don't be a drag. Don't be a party-pooper. It'll help cheer you up. You can't mope around for days on end. And I'll be mad if you break our date.

I know my friend meant well and she wanted to help. She wanted to do something—for herself, just as much as for him. She wanted to pat herself on the shoulder for being the friend in need, the one who cheered him up! She didn't want to do the hard work, quiet talk and comforting, which would be draining for her and in all likelihood would receive less fanfare. She preferred an evening of "partying"—fun with an additional bonus of assuaging her guilt.

Another story:

There were two women, Statia and Loretta, who were very close. Both were married and had families. Loretta was a housewife but Statia had recently returned to work; she had been very successful and was working with a large international firm. One day there was terrible news: Loretta's husband had been killed in a car accident. Statia was in her office when she heard, and she was shocked. Her first thought was for Loretta. "My God— how awful. She must be grief-stricken. I wonder what I should do . . . what can I do?" But she couldn't think of anything, and she finally sat down to write her best friend a condolence letter! As she did so, a colleague of hers, a Spanish man who worked for the firm, entered the room and listened as she explained her dilemma, ending her story with, "and I just don't know how to help her. I don't know what to do."

"What to do? What to do?" the Spaniard exclaimed in bewilderment. "Go to her, go to her; that's what we do!"

Cultural differences. I know that an Israeli would respond as the Spaniard did—"Go to her, be with her." I remembered the young boys who went to sit with the parents of a fallen fellow soldier. They would travel for hours, to sit with them. That's what it was called: sitting with them. It is a comfort, but the sitter does not take credit; it is inappropriate, for the loss of a son cannot be assuaged with flowers or flattery. Death, especially sudden death, is a part of life there. People deal with it more directly, simply because they have to. Here we are more fortunate and have the luxury of pretending it will never intrude in so ugly a way on our lives. As a result death often becomes unmentionable, "the pornography of our times." Death and illness don't mesh with the stereotypical American way of life, the ideology of rugged individualism, picking yourself up by your bootstraps, even a boy born in a log cabin can be president. Most of us don't believe external or uncontrollable events can determine our lives—they merely present the challenges. Hell, we conquered a whole continent. Not to mention the youth culture, Coca-Cola, and jogging: no room for death there. And there's the American concept of privacy—zealousness for one's own, respect for one's neighbor's. The American dream is a private home with a big yard, ostensibly for children to play in, but also as an unofficial boundary, a no-man's land to keep the neighbors at bay. We're wary of intruding. Grief, mourning, and illness are so emotional, so intimate—we immediately assume others want privacy. People are too scared even to ask, "Would you like us to come, or would you rather be alone?" People seem terrified of communication, of talking. Yet it is those assumptions made unilaterally ("They want to be alone") which come across as rejection and retreat. We joke about it sometimes. "What do they think we're doing, that we want to be alone so much—sit around and tell each other secrets for two years?"

"We sit here and talk about why we're alone," Leora kids.

Fear of death is a universal mortal fear. Ernest Becker says it is so great that we are continually and constantly repressing it in order to function, yet still it seeps out and controls many of our actions, one of which is to shrink from illness, decay, destruction— all symbols of our own mortality.

There's another factor. Most of us have a touch of xenophobia. We all feel more comfortable with those who are similar and familiar to us. We congregate in groups based on age, marital status, sometimes religious or professional affiliation, ethnic background. We have more in common with those like us, and they don't threaten us. We don't have to fear saying the wrong thing, displaying ignorance, acting inappropriately or foolishly. But illness is neither similar nor familiar to the healthy. It is alien and frightening.

Besides, illness is an eyesore. It doesn't fit. Wheelchairs stick out; they don't blend.

January 16

We made Dad get in the wheelchair tonight. He was tired, and falling all over the place. We insisted that he start using the wheelchair in the evenings on a regular basis. He agreed. I didn't realize how much it upset him, but to him it had great significance. He wanted to know the exact date. Sixteenth or seventeenth, I said, why? It's the first day I really had to get in a wheelchair, he said, I want to remember.

"It's weird," he said. "I mean, you tell your muscles to work and they don't listen. You say to your left leg: 'move!' And it moves, an eighth of an inch. And you say to your right leg: 'move!' And it doesn't move at all. So you turn back to your left leg. 'Move!' . . . I was always scared of this disease. Way before I had it. Of all other illnesses. I remember watching a baseball game on TV—this was in the Sixties, when we were in Baltimore—and some Yanks got on and talked about the Gehrig Foundation. They were trying to raise money for research. I got so angry, I snapped the TV off. I was mad. I was mad at them for reminding me that the disease existed. I was mad because they made me think about it."

Mom and Dana had gotten him in bed and we were all sitting around, talking and hugging him, he telling us to support each other. The wheelchair was a white flag to him, the beginning of the end.

There's a quotation in a psychiatric paper by a Dr. Jerry Holland, of something a woman with cancer told her psychiatrist. "This disease isn't just killing me, doctor," she said, "it's destroying my whole family." That isn't happening in our family. We're still living. We talk about it when we have to, but we don't dwell on it. We also talk about Begin's meshugas and the Moral Majority and Reaganomics. And we kid Dad: "Are you urinating in the living room again, Dad?" If you don't laugh at life, life will laugh at you.

February 1982

David has had some extended conversations with Dr. Fitzgerald lately. He told him he was disappointed that he hadn't made a point of staying in touch on a regular basis. Initially Fitzgerald responded by saying that it never occurred to him David would want him to do so, but of course it had, because Pauline had conveyed the request. She had run into him at a conference and he had commented that he hadn't seen David in several months, how was he? "Why don't you give him a ring—I know he'd appreciate it," Mom had suggested. But later in the conversation Fitzgerald said he felt awkward doing it—it had crossed his mind several times but each time he would get caught up in things and forget. David believed the part about the awkwardness, but told Fitzgerald that he didn't understand how the awkwardness could outweigh and overrun not only the potential comfort to the sufferer, but the humanistic and Hippocratic duty to stay in touch with a chronically ill individual.

Still, David learned an important lesson for physicians from Ftzgerald. Fitzgerald had said that he never knew quite what his role was—friend, physician, or mere acquaintance. That David had come to see him in the first place expressed implicit confidence and trust in him as a physician, but David was well versed in neurology himself and he had sought opinions elsewhere, though he always told his consultants that he had a doctor in Nashville, and always had Fitzgerald's encouragement and foreknowledge. How should Fitzgerald have acted? David's advice to doctors in this predicament is to communicate with the patient: "Let's clarify our roles. I don't know how to relate to you. How would it be most comfortable to you?"

David was also upset by a careless remark Fitzgerald had once made. "You say I have difficulty accepting my dependency needs," David told him. "Well, who doesn't? Especially when they increase every day. But I do accept them. You don't know what enables me to sit here wearing a shirt and trousers. A wheelchair is trivial in comparison. You don't know how I pass water, or who wipes my backside. So you see, that was a very hurtful statement you made, it hurt me and the family. You don't know what my dependency needs are. You don't know who takes care of me, and what they have to do for me. You're in a difficult position and I realize that—you think you have nothing to offer me because you have no treatment. But you can offer support. You see, a trivial statement for you is very hurtful to us. What amazes me, I guess, is that you haven't stayed in touch with me out of intellectual curiosity, if nothing else. You know the quote from Sir William Osler: 'To study the phenomena of disease without books is to sail an uncharted sea, while to study books without patients is not to go to sea at all.' You don't know ALS. You only know it from the textbooks. You don't know the disease. Pauline knows ALS. My family knows ALS. George knows ALS. They know the changes it brings over the months. They know the difference between me in November and me in January. They know the time I lost my legs but still had my arms. They know the time I lost my arms but still had my hands. They know when I lost my hands and couldn't write anymore. They knew when I could still put on my clothes; now I have to be dressed. They knew when I could bathe myself; now it's a whole procedure. They're experts in ALS. Here you have the opportunity to work with an intelligent individual who's facing his disease in a cerebral and level-headed manner, and you haven't tried to learn the practical aspects of the disease from him—for the sake of the people you could help cope with this illness in the future."

When Dad relayed this conversation he said those were the harshest words he had even spoken to Fitzgerald. Fitzgerald had nothing to say in return.

Today Dad just about hit the roof. Dr. Kaye called. Just back from a big medical conference in New Orleans, and he told Dad, "Several people asked about your health and sent regards, but I can't remember who the hell they were."

That's the worst thing about the Kayes. People still think of them as "some of the Rabins' closest friends." They flock to Ted and Sally to ask how we are and send regards. But the good words and kind wishes—"Please tell him I'm thinking about him," "I'm a terrible letter writer but I'd love to visit him—Does he receive visitors?"—never reach us.

Sometimes I think we get so obsessed with the people stuff because it's easier. It's manageable. Man-made. Maybe we can even triumph. Unlike the illness, which is elusive and uncontrollable, mysterious.

Yet we are becoming so bogged down in it. It's draining us. Sometimes I feel like boarding up the house against the hostile world, nailing wooden planks across the windows and posting "No Entry" signs, turning out the lights.

Late February

Dad is very depressed. His arms have become so thin they are like wrists; his feet are swollen like a grandmother's, the ankles drowned in mounds of flesh. All day on his seat, with no fat left for padding. We turn him, we rearrange his legs, bend his knees, worry about our backs. And all the time, his muscles are twitching, jumping, ticking, clicking, tweaking. No peace. They shoot horses, don't they? His words. Sometimes his speech is so slow and slurred we finish the sentence for him, just to get it over with. Or he makes faces, nodding or contorting his mouth to express mockery, disbelief, endorsement, bewilderment, or a request for more information. I realize now why he gave those monologues; he had things he wanted to get said.

"How much does he have to suffer?" Mom asks. "How much must any one human being suffer?" But that implies a reason or an order there cannot be. Some mornings he sobs at the prospect of facing another day. When we hold him it makes it harder for him to stop. "Don't, don't," he shakes his head emphatically as we approach, and we back off cautiously. And he tries to smile, raising his eyebrows and baring his big white teeth.

And all the time his mind is racing, running, galloping away but held back on a string. Like a yo-yo cut short, or a child's wind-up motor car which keeps hitting its front against the wall getting nowhere, the wheels spinning in place, a two-wheel drive stuck in mud. Whenever I see those stuck toys I want to pick them up quickly and set them free, let them go.

And Leora says to me, "There's a superstition: if a bird flies into the house there's going to be a death there. And there are blackbirds trying to get in upstairs. You can hear them banging their beaks against the sides of the house in the laundry room. They keep trying to get in but they can't. Go up there, you'll hear them." I tell her she's crazy and that that is silly, but I go up out of curiosity. I hear them, crashing against the walls of our fortress.

Drag my feet and stop time. This we can handle but the worst is yet to come. Mom shows me the aspirator, a machine with a suction tube, in case Dad chokes on a piece of cheese or a slug of orange juice. It has to be plugged in, so we go out and get a nine-foot-long extension cord. It's no guarantee because sometimes there's no morsel in Dad's throat, he's just having a spasm and can't catch his breath. "This is the way a lot of people with ALS die." Mom takes me in the bathroom, shows me where to place the tube on his tongue, down his throat right-in-the-middle, as far down as you can go. Then she closes the door. "You have to realize—many die this way. Know that ahead of time—it's not your fault."

We are careful. We've gotten none of the winter flus and viruses. As soon as we feel achy we go upstairs, take an aspirin and are quarantined, straight to bed. If people who visit feel something coming on they let us know and cancel. We've been lucky— knock on wood. There's only so much we can do. Mom says,

"Whenever something happened, I said to myself, 'We'll get over this somehow.' This, we'll never get over."

Widow. An awful word. Even "widower" seems to carry more respect. Like the difference between "cripple" and "disabled." I remember a column by Ellen Goodman on the death of spouses called "Women Mourn, Men Replace." She offered explanations. "Maybe women believe too much in uniqueness. [Or perhaps it is that] women wallow, men act." Mom says that above all she'll miss the championship. "We'll be watching something on TV, not saying a word, and all of a sudden I'll look up and say, 'This is awful!' And he'll say, 'Yes, turn it off.' He's my rock of Gibraltar."

Sometimes Mom gets angry and bitter, and Dad seems to entrust me with words for her. "You can be supportive to her without getting hung up on her neuroses. Your mother is an excellent psychiatrist. She's got a very good job here but even if it falls through and she doesn't get tenure . . . after all, I brought her to Nashville but she could get a job anywhere. If she says she's too old to get a new job or not qualified enough—that's nonsense. You have to remind her: she's good. She doesn't always remember. She didn't get the Vanderbilt position because she's my wife—she got it on her own. Right now she feels hurt by many of her colleagues and many of our friends in the community. But that would have happened anywhere we had lived with a certain percentage of the people. You have to remember that. You and Mom are alike—you can be happy or miserable anywhere if you make up your mind to. Don't lose faith in people though. There are good and bad people everywhere. So be optimistic—don't be Pollyannaish; be realistic; but be positive."

Mom's like the little girl with the curl. When she's good she's very very good, she's tough as nails. But when she's down she's down and out. She says we're so unlucky—except for the kids, such wonderful kids she has, she's lucky. But Daddy's so wasted, just skin and bones; he can't even hold her anymore. And he worries we'll remember him that way—a bag of bones. Demanding, tiresome, sick, always sick.

"But he's not—he's my source of strength," she says. "He's my rock of Gibraltar, even if he just sits there." Sometimes he helps her on the nephrology book she's editing. "I can't do anymore," she whines. "Don't you start that again," he says. Then when he's depressed or starts crying she kids him out of it. "Oh, no you don't," and he snaps out of it. "Dad, go ahead and cry if you want to," I say, me of the in-touch-with-your-feelings generation. "No, it's unproductive," he says. "Crying is not productive and I'm not going to do it. I did enough of it last week."

Late at night Pauline talks to me. Sometimes she can't sleep, she's so afraid, so we stay up and watch bad movies half-heartedly. How to choose a husband: He must have a sense of humor. Right. No, really. "Look at Daddy: he can still laugh, even now when he's suffering so much. It makes it bearable. Will you remember Dad jogging with you, that winter in the snow? Love of life, that's another thing I suppose. For a husband. Don't laugh at me. It's important to discuss these things—they're never discussed. No wonder people make mistakes. How do you choose the person you'll spend the rest of your life with? And how else could we have made it through this? David's such a source of strength to me, even when he just sits there. I don't know what we'll do without him. You know, he says his favorite time of the day is the mornings, on the weekends, when we stay in bed and cuddle. He's good to cuddle with."

Sometimes I wonder who I worry about the most. Dana, who walks around with her head covered in a cloud of sun dust, an intricate screening and filtering mechanism. She keeps everything tidy, picture-perfect; a defense against chaos. Her job is the laundry, and every evening a batch arrives on your bed, shirts folded with their arms back like they should; even the socks pair up. When I look a number up in the phone book she snatches it and puts it back on the shelf before I've had a chance to dial. David is flawless in her eyes, but he keeps reminding her: just because I'm sick doesn't mean I'm always right, I'm not perfect, you know. It's dangerous to think someone's perfect—you discover flaws later on and the whole image cracks into smithereens, such disappointment. "Don't you worry!" Dana turns around, surprising all of us. Gives him a rundown: "First of all, you've been losing your temper lately. You correct us for little things like bad table manners, and you don't realize how much you upset people when you do that. I don't think you're perfect! What a nerve! Another thing is, you want me to be a doctor.

And I know you think it's a good, secure profession and that makes you happy, but I don't want to be a doctor. I want to be a teacher, and work with handicapped children. I enjoyed it when I did it last summer. Besides, I hate biology and chemistry even though I'm good at them. You're a snob about professions; you want us all to be doctors and lawyers. . . ."

We all have our roles. Dana is the dreamer, Dad is the rock, and I'm the *littérateur*; when everyone gets mad that people talk about us, I remind them what Oscar Wilde said: "There is only one thing in the world worse than being talked about, and that is not being talked about."

And Leora—she's a toughie. You don't mess with Leora. Sometimes she's so tough you forget she's just a kid. Like the first time she brushed Dad's teeth. He has a big gap where three molars are missing, from the days of Aliwal North in South Africa when the doctor's cure-all was to pull teeth. Leora thought it was recent, part of the illness. So she brushed only his front teeth. "Hey, what're you doing?" he asked her. "Oh, I thought you didn't have any teeth back there. . . ." But she's perceptive. One day she was upset and I was trying to soothe her. "We're okay, we're managing," I said. "But don't you see? We'll only really get over it after Daddy dies." Or as Dad puts it: "This crisis will only be resolved one way, and that's by another crisis."

Leora calls Dad "Pops." "What's up, Pops?" And she gets mad when he says, "Not much." He agrees with her. He should think of something new to say; ill people become myopic.

She didn't tell us when she strained her back helping Dad. Stayed in her room until noon one Sunday; finally we had to go in to find out what was going on. Sometimes she freaks out— she's got lots of energy and guts and vivacity. Wants to go out and boogie and sneak beer into parties and get caught and run away and cruise around in Robert's Yellow Banana and be like everybody else. Quietly she worries about money. "This time next year we'll be in Calcutta," she slips out to me. "God, no," I say. "We've got insurance and money put away and Mom'll still be bringing in a salary." I go talk to Dad, tell him he should explain to her in detail, money and figures, it's probably eating her up.

* * *

Michael was home for a few weeks. It's very hard for him. Thinking he should be here, to help with an extra hand. When he's here he takes over duties with Dad. "Here, this is how we do it. Easier that way—hold his back, there." Michael cringes at every "we," a reminder of his being apart from us. Maybe they were wrong to keep him in the dark for so long. But right now he's looking for a summer job in Nashville. There isn't much.

He told me something that worried me. "No one listens to me," Michael said. "Dana and Leora don't take my advice. I tell them I'm older; I've had experience. You don't listen to me either. Not like you listen to Dad. Who's going to replace him when he's gone if you don't listen to me?"

Whoa! "You *can't* try to replace him," I told him. "You shouldn't even try. Anyway, it's not as if we listen to his advice all the time. And before he got sick—think about it. No one can replace him, Michael. I can't, you can't, Mom can't. Don't even try. You're crazy. You'll never succeed, not like you'd want, and you'll feel you failed him. Anyway, it'd be artificial. It's impossible. You better get that idea out of your head. It's dangerous. When he's gone, that's it. He's gone."

"There's got to be some way to keep his courage—his spirit—alive. There's got to."

"The challenge will be to keep the family alive as a unit and a community."

"That's what's amazing. We've stayed together. Look at all the families that crumble over trivialities. Remember the family that lived in the apartment above us in Jerusalem? They moved out—she had lung cancer, and she couldn't climb the stairs? He remarried as soon as she died; he'd been having an affair the whole time. Everyone knew it. I thought it was awful to hurt her like that, when she was already suffering so much."

"Mom said she could understand. He needed support, and why should his life be cut off? But Mom—look at her. She's totally devoted to Dad. She's still in love with him. I guess the difference is that he supports her. He isn't just a drain."

"That's what I mean. Y'know, one day I was real depressed—well, it happens a lot up at school. I don't have any motivation to work and I say to myself: What the hell am I doing here? Anyway, I was going to go see *Chariots of Fire*—it's supposed to be a really motivating movie. Before I went I was going to call home. So I called and changed my mind about going to the movie. I talked to Dad. He could tell something was wrong. He said, 'You've got a job to do, Mike. I'm doing my job down here. You do yours too.' That was all the motivation I needed to hear. It was like a hot poker."

Keeping the courage alive.

"That's going to be our heritage, Michael."

March 1982

We've called for David's brother Tots to come.

He told us months ago he was on standby for us; now we need him. Dad is requiring more and more care and we can't handle it all ourselves. At least, that's what we say. What we are scared to admit is that we need someone to come. Not to do anything, just to be here. An outsider who is willing to come inside.

We throw out ideas about how we will handle the new burdens that are added every day. Mom says she will quit her job, make arrangements to work at home. The first is out of the question. It's not only a question of finances. More than that, Mom simply needs to get out of the house and continue being her own person. She can't afford to become a slave to David's needs.

The family in South Africa seems closer now. Mom let it slip that David needed to gain weight and loved the South African chocolates: Kit Kats and flaky Aeros and white creamy chocolate. Now cartonfuls of the stuff arrive regularly. Not one or two mailings—constant deliveries. They come faster than we can consume them, and that's pretty fast. We've begun freezing them. Soon the basement freezer will overflow; we'll have to give the precious things away. Other goodies come too: Milo, a chocolate milk powder supplemented with vitamins; anchovy paste, as salty as it sounds; and Byrd's Eye Custard powder, a delicious instant pudding, protein and dessert in one.

Letters come too. Sweet, gossipy letters from Joyce, cryptic letters from Tots written in script even he cannot understand. Notes from Jack scribbled on the back of picture postcards of zebras and lions in the game reserves. Long hilarious letters from our cousin Sharon, whose exploits at college read like a comic strip.

And then there are the phone calls. The phone calls are the hardest. Transatlantic calls usually are. Keeping your eye glued to the clock, speaking in generalities, screaming to be heard when the subject matter dictates whispering. Not being able to see when the subject dictates holding. But the main reason the phone calls are difficult is because the family wants to hear something we cannot tell them: that David is getting better. That it was all a horrible mistake. That it had been a false alarm, and now there's nothing to worry about. If not that, at least that he's making progress, on his way to recovery. But we can't say that. "He's holding his own," Mom says. "I'm hanging in there," Dad says. And sometimes, Mom, "Well, he's not been doing so well. He's had some setbacks lately."

He's had a bit of a setback. He seems to be stabilizing. Well, you know with this disease you don't really get better, you just hope you'll get worse slowly; and he seems to be getting worse slowly.

Tots must have flinched inwardly when he saw Dad the first time, but he never showed it. He acted as though the tears in his eyes were the normal tears of any blood reunion. Tots knows David; knows the last thing his little brother wants is pity or sadness. We all kissed and hugged and felt a queer relief. We had been joined by another one of us. We thought we had reached the end of the line, only to turn around and find others there behind us.

I really never knew Tots until now. I realize I had kept the image my parents portrayed of him during his youth. Spontaneous. Impetuous. Sometimes a little wild. The image appealed to me. I stuck to it even though Dad warned me Tots was different, older and wiser, a married man with two grown-up daughters. Now I see the real Tots, neither their image nor my own. A man who has made himself a nurse to my father. A man to whom illness has been only a distant mystery in the past has transformed himself into a gentle nurse, cook, and companion. He taught himself how to cook an egg for David in the morning, mix a tunafish salad for him at lunch. How to spread the newspaper out for him. How to hold him just so as he picks him up out of the bed. They spend the mornings reviewing the printed galleys of David's book, checking meticulously for errors and typos. Over lunch they discuss the racial situation in South Africa, the tensions in the Middle East. Late in the afternoon they slip into closed door sessions during which they talk about darker things—the future, wills, financial arrangements. In the evenings we stay home, watching television and catching up on the family characters. Nothing is forced. Everything is as it should be. He's family and he feels one of us, one with us.

Tots is leaving today. Thank God Joyce is supposed to get here just two weeks from now. This is lucky. I think Dad would be very depressed otherwise, but now he has something to look forward to. Another shipment of reinforcements is coming in.

Joyce is different, gentle and soft. Secretly, I suppose, we expected her to cry uncontrollably when she came. But she didn't. She had been warned not to, and waited until afterward when she was safely stowed away in her room washing for dinner. Joyce is a lady. She moves gracefully, avoids speaking politics, never raises her voice. She brought with her a suitcase full of gifts, and beams when we come down wearing the embroidered sweaters and African skirts. She bakes constantly, filling the house with the smells of rising muffins, cinnamon buns, and sweet bread. She makes custard for David, casseroles for dinner. And every Friday night two loaves of braided challahs, over which she stands, covers her eyes with her hands and blesses the candles precisely at sunset. Every time we walk in the door from school or work she is ready with a cup of hot tea and a warm cookie straight from the oven. No admonitions for us to refrain from gobbling too many—she wants us to eat. She is cooking for us, nourishing us; feeding us, nurturing us.

Joyce is an amazing storyteller. She can go on for hours, relaying story after story, each with pithy endings that wrap everything up in neat little packages making sensible orders of the world. How she re-met her high school boyfriend, twenty-five years later. Or how the woman, who had had an affair for years, finally divorced her husband for her beau and then got dumped. Or how the people who tried to sneak gold Krugerrands out of South Africa in brassieres got caught in customs. Or how they finally discovered why the family down the street had acted so strangely for years. The family had been a pillar in the community to whom everyone had always looked up. But then the father took ill and it became like a different family. Such a tragedy. Even in the best of families.

I think now that we are just one story in a string of stories, all tied together, making sense not individually but as a piece of a pattern. Like a walletful of snapshots, glimpses of the human story.

Our story. Our obligation to tell it.

August 1982

This is the article as it appeared in the *New England Journal of Medicine*, 19 August 1982:

It has been three years since my first symptoms suggested a diagnosis of amyotrophic lateral sclerosis (ALS). The pain and anguish of this illness are known to most physicians and are an inevitable accompaniment of the disease, but there are other unpleasant aspects that are avoidable. In this article I want to relate my personal story and to emphasize the extraordinary change that my illness brought about in my interrelations with fellow physicians.

I turned 45 in January 1979. I was then director of endocrinology at the Vanderbilt Medical Center, and my research in the areas of metabolism and reproduction was flourishing. I was supremely happy with my wife and family; we traveled often and enjoyed an active and varied social life. My wife and I had both graduated from the University of Witwatersrand in Johannesburg, South Africa. After completing our postgraduate education at Johns Hopkins Medical Center, we had stayed on the faculty for nearly a decade. We then spent five years in Israel working at the Hadassah Medical Center, and in 1975 we returned to the States and settled in Nashville.

My years at Vanderbilt have been very happy. The foundation for this happiness is the atmosphere of unusual cordiality and collegiality that is the hallmark of this medical school. I had known the rampant political intrigues of the academic world and had found them abhorrent, but at Vanderbilt there is a spirit of cooperation and collaboration that makes going to work a pleasure. Politics always exist in an intellectual and competitive environment. What is unique about Vanderbilt is the choice it offers to eschew such distractions and concentrate on the fundamentals of one's profession. As a result, my years here have been characterized by academic advancement, many friendships, and a sense of acceptance by students, house staff, and colleagues. This background is important to the story I am about to relate because, whereas I had previously been "at" Hopkins and "at" Hadassah, I now felt I was "of" Vanderbilt.

During my early years at medical school I had steeped myself in the study of neurologic anatomy and had shown precocious talent in clinical neurology. I did not choose neurology, however. My reasons were clear: the diagnostic problem seemed largely an academic exercise—so little, if anything, could be done for the patient in a definitive therapeutic way. The years, as well as my own illness, however, have taught me how wrong it is to focus on definitive therapy and how much can and should be done for the patient, even when one is confronted with so-called incurable illness. In any event, although my field became endocrinology, my knowledge of neurology did not evaporate. How nice this would turn out to be. In June of 1979 I noticed some stiffness in my legs. Within two short weeks I discovered quite by chance that my reflexes had become pathologically brisk. When I could no longer dismiss fasciculation as mere "restless legs" and it became clear that there were no sensory symptoms, the diagnosis of ALS reached my consciousness despite every attempt at denial.

This story will confine itself to the effects of my illness on my relationship with my fellow physicians—whether they were my personal physicians, professional colleagues, or old friends. My strategy was to avoid disclosure of my illness for as long as possible, for the following reasons. First of all, my wife and I agreed that ignorance was a blessing, especially for our children who would eventually have to endure with us the pain and suffering of a progressive, inexorable decline in my health. Secondly, even though I had and still have the greatest regard for my colleagues and know that the respect, affection, and admiration are mutual, I realized intuitively that their knowledge of my illness could destroy my professional life at the medical center.

Let me share some of the reactions of my professional colleagues, beginning with an account of the behavior of my personal physician. To confirm the diagnosis, I traveled to a prestigious medical center renowned for its experience with ALS. The diagnostic and technical skills of the people there were superb, and more than matched the reputation of the institution. The neurologist was rigorous in his examination and deft in reaching an unequivocal diagnosis. My disappointment stemmed from his impersonal manner. He exhibited no interest in me as a person, and did not make even a perfunctory inquiry about my work. He gave me no guidelines about what I should do, either concretely—in terms of daily activities—or, what was more important, psychologically, to muster the emotional strength to cope with a progressive degenerative disease. Stetten recently described his experience after receiving a diagnosis of progressive macular degeneration: "No ophthalmologist has mentioned any of the many ways in which I could stem the deterioration in the quality of my life."[1] The only thing my doctor did offer me was a pamphlet setting out in grim details the future that I already knew about too well. He asked to see me in three months, and I was too polite or too cowed to ask him why— what benefit was there for me to make the journey again? I still recall that the only time he seemed to come alive during our interview was when he drew the mortality curve among his collected patients for me. "Very interesting," he said. "There's a break in the slope after three years." When, a few months later, I read an article by him in which he emphasized the importance of a compassionate and supportive role for the physician caring for the patient with ALS, I wondered whether he had been withdrawn because I was a physician.

By the fall of 1979 I was walking with a limp; I countered the queries I received in every corridor by saying that I had "a disk." This was not threatening to my colleagues, who proffered advice on how to deal with it and regaled me with their own back problems. I was still a full member of the fraternity, in excellent standing. By early 1980, however, the limp was worse, and I now held a cane in my right hand.

[1] Stetten, D., Jr. "Coping with Blindmen." *New England Journal of Medicine* 305 (1981): 458–60.

The inquiries ceased and were replaced by a very obvious desire to avoid me. When I arrived at work in the morning I could see, from the corner of my eye, colleagues changing their pace or stopping in their tracks to spare themselves the embarrassment of bumping into me. This dramatic change in their behavior occurred when it became common knowledge that David Rabin had ALS. I state with total conviction that my colleagues never meant to hurt me. On the contrary, I was *of* Vanderbilt, and they grieved for me, yet were unable to express their grief.

As the cane became inadequate and was replaced by a walker, so my isolation from my colleagues intensified. I recognize that my own behavior and personality may have contributed to the situation: I am gregarious and, I believe, warm with people; I also value my independence. I did not call a press conference to announce that I had ALS; I did not raise a banner asking for help; rather, I continued to do my work insofar as I was able. Did that put them off? Did they reason, "He wants to pretend that everything is normal, so let's play his game"? How often, as I struggled to open a door, would I see a colleague pretending to look the other way? On the other hand, why was it so natural for the nonphysicians—the technicians, the secretaries, the cleaning women—to rush to open the door for me, even if it was the door to the men's toilet? I can only guess that my colleagues thought it would embarrass me if they offered help. How wrong they were, and how distorted their reasoning—accepting help is preferable to sustaining a fracture.

One day, while crossing the little courtyard outside the emergency room, I fell. A longtime colleague was walking by. He turned, and our eyes met as I lay sprawled on the ground. He quickly averted his eyes, pretended not to see me, and continued walking. He never even broke his stride. I suppose he ignored the obvious need for help out of embarrassment and discomfort, for I know him to be a compassionate and caring physician. In trying to understand the behavior of my colleagues I recall an experience I had when I was at Hopkins. I had worked with a splendid physician, Dr. Mason Lord. While still young he developed a brain tumor, and he lingered for six or seven months. I always thought up a dozen good reasons to avoid visiting him. Finally, I convinced myself that he really wanted to see only his close friends and family. Of course, I was merely rationalizing. We knew and liked each other, and I failed to go to see him because I would be uncomfortable—not he. I remember my sense of futility when I attended his funeral, because by then it was too late to comfort Mason Lord.

There are so many ways colleagues can help a sick physician. I have learned that the Vanderbilt community admired my ability to continue, in spite of my illness, to function, to maintain my lecture schedule, to write grants and have them awarded, to write papers and have them accepted. The school established an annual lectureship in my name, and my family and I were very moved by this expression of respect and acknowledgment. In the light of this, I may seem ungrateful, and my sense of isolation may seem unwarranted. Nonetheless, continuing personal contact with my colleagues has been rare. I have been working at home for the past year—an arrangement made possible through the consistent and unflagging support of my department chairman. A group of physicians, nurses, and technicians come on a regular basis to work with me. But very few of the physicians with whom I am not collaborating have either called, written, or come to visit.

Some of my close relationships with fellow physicians have also deteriorated since my illness. For a friend to maintain interest and empathy for a week or a month was relatively easy; to show sustained concern over three years required a commitment of quite a different order. I have received relatively few telephone calls or letters from the scores of colleagues I have met in more than twenty years of academic life: former fellows and students, fellow members of study section, faculty members at numerous medical schools where I have lectured. I hear indirectly about their concern, however, the definitive step of writing me a letter of support is more than the majority can manage. Why this deafening silence? Perhaps it is because we, as physicians, are the healers. We dispense treatment, counsel, and support; and we represent strength. The dichotomy of being both doctor and patient threatens the integrity of the club. To this fraternity of healers, becoming ill is tantamount to treachery. Furthermore, the sick physician makes us uncomfortable. He reminds us of our own vulnerability and mortality, and this is frightening for those of us who deal with disease every day while arming ourselves with an imagined cloak of immunity against personal illness.

We can all recall times when we stood by while a fellow physician behaved irrationally or became frankly psychotic. Most of us are aware of colleagues who are abusing alcohol or drugs. Usually, we delicately ignore the obvious until disaster overtakes the unfortunate physician. I was glad to read in a recent issue of the *Journal* that Vanderbilt is taking steps to help alcoholic physicians.[2] I remember a sensitive and capable psychiatrist at Hopkins who was subject to manic-depressive episodes. His colleagues and I observed the development of manic behavior. We did not intervene, and shortly thereafter his body was found hanging from the ceiling in his hospital office.

It would be erroneous and unfair to say that all physicians avoid and neglect their sick colleagues. In my own case, there are several who have been doggedly and unflinchingly helpful to my family and me. "You have the illness," one friend told me, "but we are in this together." He meant it, and he has followed through with action consistently, to this very day. Although he has a family, a thriving practice, and many interests, he never hides behind the screen of a busy schedule. It has been the thoughtfulness, concern, and spontaneity of many people like him that has enabled my family and me to face the trials and sorrows of this disease. In fact, some physicians with whom we had very little contact before the illness have come forward in our time of need. There are close friends who live many miles away, yet make the time and incur the expense of coming to visit us frequently. One of my former fellows actually moved into my home and helped me in all kinds of ways, including getting me to and from work for eight months.

This account is not intended as a litany of complaint but as a call to physicians to express the compassion they feel toward sick colleagues. It is also meant to draw attention to our frequent inability as physicians to deal with members of our profession who no longer fit the mold of the compleat healer. Toward these ends, I would like to make some concrete suggestions. First of all, do not ignore your colleague. Greet him. Inquire about his health. Offer him support if he

[2] Spickard, A., and Billings, F.T., Jr. "Alcoholism in a Medical School Faculty." *New England Journal of Medicine* 305 (1981): 1646–48.

is physically handicapped. Don't assume that he prefers seclusion. Ask to visit him. Don't hide behind the false morality of "respecting his privacy"; if it is inconvenient he will tell you.

Secondly, be conscious of the family and extend your support to them. Make a point of asking how your colleague's spouse is feeling and how he or she is coping. The spouse and the children are suffering at least as much as the victim and need support, encouragement, and acknowledgment of their travail. Do not expose the wife to the "premature-widow syndrome," as some physicians do who encounter my wife and never mention my name or inquire about me at all.

Thirdly, bear in mind that the absence of a magic potion against the disease does not render the physician impotent. There are many avenues that can be helpful for the victim and his family. I am often surprised and moved by the acts of kindness and affection that people perform. Fundamentally, what the family needs is the sense that people care. No one else can assume the burden, but knowing that you are not forgotten does ease the pain.

A few weeks after publication:

The response has been overwhelming. Almost as if the world has been waiting for precisely this article to be written—as if the ideas have been standing out there ripe and ready and waiting for just the right person to come along and pluck them. We have received five hundred letters, and they're still coming in. From everybody: colleagues of David's. Other people with neurologic disorders and terminal illness. People we know. Total strangers. People who apologized because they had behaved that way themselves. People who were victims of the behavior we described. And everybody thanked us for finally saying it, for taking it out of the closet, for educating them. We read the letters, cry over them, savor them. The message is loud and clear: You are not alone. You are right to feel hurt and you are brave to protest. David answers each one personally.

A former student of David tells of her visit home to her terminally ill mother during medical school. When she returned to campus, hoping to collapse into the arms of supportive friends, she found only rejection, confusion, and coldness resulting from an inability to communicate.

A woman whose husband died of a terrible brain-damaging disease said lifelong friends of the family never even acknowledged the death. Just never mentioned it.

An ALS patient described how she had confided her condition to her best friend of twelve years. "I never heard from her again," she wrote. "I feel like I have leprosy."

The director of a cancer institute wrote saying the article confirmed what he had seen and heard expressed time and time again from other cancer patients.

"What you described is exactly what happened to my husband— the averted eyes, the embarrassment."

"I know exactly what you are talking about. It happened to my sister."

"My mother had the same thing happen to her. I still think it was that, and not the disease, that killed her."

"It happened to me."

"It happened to my best friend."

"I have been guilty of it. I vow I will never do it again."

People drew analogies to other kinds of tragic situations. A former alcoholic said the most devastating consequence of her condition was the "careful avoidance" of friends and colleagues. A man whose son-in-law drowned three months after the wedding described the loneliness and isolation his daughter experienced among her college classmates. One man experienced it while going through a painful divorce. Another experiences it daily with her young son, who has cerebral palsy. Another with her young daughter, who suffers a rare stomach ailment.

The article has opened up communication for many friends. In a sense it was a beckoning, a cry, an open letter to the world. Friends had a chance to express their love and admiration.

"There have been few days since I found out about the illness when I have not thought of you. But I wondered: Would you want to see me, to hear from me. And: What would I say, how would I talk with you with your illness (as I imagined it) between us. I looked away."

Another friend wrote: "It is hard to find the words to write to you. I have been guilty of placing my discomfort ahead of your need for comfort."

A physician who used to work with David and now lives in Montana said he and other mutual friends often discuss getting in touch, "but we never did anything about it."

We see the botches of miscommunication. A former Vanderbilt medical student said her first impulse, when she learned of the illness, was to write or call. "But I was told in no uncertain terms the illness was not a topic for discussion. And you were quoted by one person as saying, 'Life is too short to talk about the things we cannot control.'"

Dad swears he never said anything even remotely resembling this.

We've seen incredible generosity from total strangers—a man who lives in Hawaii offered us the use of his home while he travels; a man with a condominium in Florida offered us a place to stay during the winter months.

And we got our share of extremists: born-again Christians promising eternal bliss. An evangelist who wrote from Malaysia. A Jew-for-Jesus.

But I think the most important thing is that people said they learned from the article. It made them stop and think. Some of Dad's endocrinologist friends have said it's his greatest contribution to medical literature. (One said it made him renew his subscription to the *Journal*.) Several medical schools are ordering reprints so they can make it mandatory reading for all faculty and students. One doctor asked for a reprint, saying, "I need it as a reminder to myself, who am in good health, for I have found excuses to put off contacts with my physician friends who have been ill. I shall also use it in my dealings with medical students for they, as I did, regard themselves as indestructible."

A neurologist said he read it and reflected upon it the next day when he had to disclose a diagnosis of ALS to a young patient. But he told her differently this time, trying to explain there was hope, and promising he would be with her along the way.

One person said he was greatly moved by the article. "After

reading it, my eyes swelled up with tears and my lips said, 'My God, Rabin, how we need you.' "

We are getting on with our lives. I just started an internship with a local newspaper and am loving it. Got a by-line the first day, when an old man nicknamed "Crip" shot and killed a truck-driver, father of six, over two hundred dollars lost in a crap game in a sleazy part of town. Luckily I got there too late to see the body—but a by-line's a by-line. Being in the newsroom is a trip: phones ringing, radio reports blaring, reporters sweating over last-minute deadlines, editors screaming and raising hell. It's a real nerve center. Always exciting; always a lot of chatter and running around. Most of the reporters are young and single; they're eager to help me out and seem to accept me as one of their own, not just a tag-along intern. We have gone out after work a couple of times—I feel back in the swing of things.

October 1982

Michael is hot on the job trail. He's in his second year of B school now—made it through the first year without "hitting the screen" (i.e., flunking out) and now he is much more relaxed, confident, and secure. He has grown much more protective, much less abashed about his love. He gloats over everything I do at the paper, nags me to send him clips so he can show off to his friends: the Rabin name in print. When he is home for the weekend the two of us slip out late at night, after putting Dad to bed, go out for a beer and share our secrets with each other in the dark corners of a bar. We talk about Dad and the family, and share notes on the state of relations between men and women. He tells me about his escapades at Harvard, where they work hard and play hard. He's made a real nice group of friends, and he tells me about their roguish exploits, skiing and sailing and weekends in Vermont. "*Goyishe nachas,*" Mom calls it. Whenever Michael comes home, and the six of us sit around, I always think what a precious thing we have here. Each one of us with his own little quirks and idiosyncrasies, always hashing and rehashing and bouncing off one another, then coming to rest together like a litter of puppies.

We're all growing up. Dana and Leora finished the last school year with shimmering report cards—Dana got straight A's, Leora all A's except for a B in gym ("Which doesn't really count," she assured us). Dana has herself a small group of friends, but she enjoys most being home with Dad, caring for him in her inimitable, gentle way. She flutters around him like a moth around light, arranging his pillows and his arms and straightening out his feet, smoothing his blanket. She's very disciplined: every day an hour is devoted to flute practice, another hour to a thin-thighs-in-thirty-days routine; several more for studying and a few sneaks at her favorite television series. Next year she'll be going to college—probably right here at Vanderbilt. It'll be a good chance for her to fly the coop a little. Mike and I are lobbying for her to live in the dorms, regardless of the situation with Dad. She should pretend Vandy is miles and miles from home, and drive in just to help once a week. She's ready for that.

Leora is different from Dana. She is running for class president and spends whole afternoons painting posterboard while Dad rhymes up snappy slogans. The classic teenager, she is learning how to drive, saving up for a stereo, always on a diet, and always on the telephone. On weekend nights she dresses to the hilt, "puts on her eyes" as Mom says, and goes out with her friends. Where are they going? Out, all over. When will they be back? Don't wait up, it'll be late for sure.

Mom, of course, got tenure at Vanderbilt. She was the only person who was surprised—naturally. She's really enjoying her teaching responsibilities, and the students pick up on that. They adore her. Just last night I went to a concert with a medical student about to start a psychiatry rotation. We ran into another student, and when he heard my friend was about to start psychiatry, he said, "Oh, you're so lucky. You'll be getting Dr. Rabin—man, she is dynamite." I started giggling and my friend explained, "This here is her daughter."

January 1983

Dad is having problems swallowing. He chokes on rice, pieces of lettuce. We give him soft mashed potatoes, pick the lettuce from his salad and leave him sliced cucumbers, tomatoes. Protein is the mainstay of his diet: white breast of chicken, diced into small pieces; boiled eggs; cottage cheese.

The clumsy green suction machine that once sat in the corner like a bad omen comes out more frequently now. We are less scared of it; even think of it as a friend. At the end of dinner he chokes, we turn and look at one another—"Should we get it?" And then one of us runs off. Usually he's recovered by the time we fetch it, find an extension cord, plug it in. Got to buy extension cords for every room in the house, Mom says. Other times we shove the mouthpiece deep into his mouth to retrieve small chunks of food and a lot of saliva.

Mom warns us again: he could choke anytime. Any one of you may be here with him when that happens. You can't feel it was your fault.

Amazing. The article has changed us.

It's funny because I don't know exactly how or why. Maybe it was the answers and their message: You're okay, you've done nothing wrong, right on. Or perhaps because by writing we have removed the cloak of shame. Before, people were hurting us, but there was such a taboo against saying anything we swallowed our hurt and anger. So we were silent, thereby giving almost tacit approval, saying to the world we deserve it, you can hit us because we're down. We were playing the victims.

Now we are proud. In a sense we have become the voice and conscience of the ill. Like in the Sixties when Black became Beautiful. Nothing to be ashamed of, we have our own beauty.

Yesterday Kate called. Gosh, I hadn't talked to her in years. I thought she must have read the article. But no: she had some work she wanted David to review. I told her I'd ask him about it. The conversation was just about to come to an end and she hadn't even asked how he was doing. Hell if I was going to hang up and then stew over it all evening. "Kate," I said quietly, "you haven't even asked how Dad is doing. You do know how sick he is, don't you?" There, I did it. "Oh, I know he's sick; that's why I didn't ask. I know he's doing so poorly," she said. "Well, that's not the only reason you ask. You ask to show concern too. Show you care, y'know." Yeah, she agreed, I was right. They think about him all the time and would really like to come and see him. I said sure, he loves having visitors, let's set up a time.

When I got off the phone they were cheering in the next room.

February 10, 1983

Today a surgeon came over. Mom and Dad closed off the living room, sat with him at the dining room table, and asked his opinion. Later they explained the options: one, a gastronomy, cutting a hole into his stomach and implanting a short plastic tube through which we would feed him on liquids. And what happens to the hole, Mom? The skin will hug up tight around it, a permanent gaping wound to be cleaned daily, rubbed with antiseptic cloths, bandaged with clear white gauze pads, and keep an eye on the infection. But Dad wants to go on eating. He says he's worried his diet will suffer and he will lose more precious weight. But I think he likes those Hershey chocolate kisses; he sucks on them and they melt smoothly down his throat.

Other surgery to consider: a tracheotomy. A hole would be punctured at the base of his neck, a clean aluminum tube inserted. How would he talk? It would cut off the air; you would have to hold your finger over the hole. How would he breathe, Mom? Through the hole. But why, what would it do, what's the advantage? It would make it easier to get into his throat and bronchi and pull out all the mucus and spit he can't get rid of on his own. If he had a tracheotomy, we would have two suction machines: one for his mouth, the other with a long, thin tube to insert into the hole, down into the bronchi to vacuum clean his airways so he can breathe.

We still have a while to go for that one, Dad says, we can put it off for now.

Later.

I can see my father: the new bionic man. Tubes dangling from his throat and stomach, wheels moving him around the room, oxygen tanks by his side just in case. Is this my father, who started jogging at age forty because he wanted to help me get in shape? My father, who was so good-looking my college friends asked me who my new boyfriend was when he came to visit? My father, with the steady hands, who always drove in the snow, jumped the battery?

He still seems to think so. Still a glint in his eye when you walk in the room, a word of encouragement, knowledge to share. Soul in a different house.

I have heard of obese men who lost pounds and pounds only to discover they miss being so big they command attention by sheer volume. My father, shrunken and weak, still radiates confidence and calm, still captures our attention. His body irrelevant, he himself a glitter of hope.

Only one thing I can't imagine. Only one thing I can't see. Only one thing would make him dead while still living—if he couldn't speak. If we were having a fight and he couldn't step in to resolve it. If he had a funny line he couldn't share. If we were arguing about the name of a composer and he knew who was right, or that all of us were wrong.

Like being bound and gagged by your own body. Like being buried alive.

March 1983

Today I came home, found a Morse code alphabet lying casually on the kitchen table. They say ALS patients can use it with their eyes because they rarely lose the muscles of the eyelids. A long blink, a short blink; two long blinks; two short and one long; three short. Christ, by the time he said "My nose itches" the itch would be gone.

We hear things. Teases. The marvels of computers; great new machines for the handicapped; talking wheelchairs. "There must be something." "They're making all kinds of technological advances these days." But how do you find out? The doctors know nothing. Even good old Susie, the occupational therapist, has no idea. Our friends in Baltimore are making inquiries and Michael is on the phone day and night. Something's on the way, he keeps hearing. There's a breakthrough just around the corner. I'm just waiting for some grant money to complete the project, they say. But we need something soon.

How frustrating. Some friends of the Cohens heard a news spot on Paul Harvey's radio show—a computer that was adapted especially for an ALS patient, lucky enough to be a computer freak's mother. It presents her with a vocabulary and alphabet and she chooses the letters by biting on a switch when the cursor reaches the appropriate one. Exactly what we need! Michael calls the radio station and gets the name Aaron Aronowitz of Maplevale, California. But there is no Aronowitz in Maplevale, there is no Maplevale. Michael calls back the station. Tries to explain: this is serious. This is exactly what we need. Time is running out, my father a brilliant scientist. . . . But to no avail: they didn't have the name; they can't disclose it. Christ, Michael says, then what's the point of doing the story?

One clue and one dead end. But at least we know it's out there somewhere.

Bull's-eye. Today we hit the jackpot. A doctor up in Chicago, who had been writing to Dad ever since the *Journal* article appeared, wrote to tell him about his marvelous new computer. The creator is—get this—Walt Waltosz, of Sunnyvale, California. He created the computer for his mother-in-law. And will soon be launching his own business, adapting computers for any and every disability. Nonprofit, or just about: for less than $3,000 we got the computer and program, along with printer and voice synthesizer and a cabinet to hold the equipment thrown into the deal. Should be here in less than two weeks, special delivery.

Late March 1983

One night we were wheeling Dad out of the room and he said, "I'm not myself any more. I loved life. Do you remember? Remember what I was like? I can hardly remember."

I try to remember. I try to see him standing or walking. He had a funny way of standing—his legs went straight down until the knee and then they splayed out, as though at odds with each other. He was in good shape. But how did he run? How did he lean over to pet the dog, or to put an arm around Mother? Images taken for granted, I never bothered to press them into memories.

I remember when I was very young, maybe six, we used to swim out past the big waves to where the sea was deep blue and quiet. He'd hold me in his arms while he did the swimming. One time, just as we had gotten out to the quiet, the lifeguards came out to get us, four or five of them. They thought we were in trouble, so far out. They must've been pretty worried, but we were fine. They had buoys and life preservers and rafts to offer me, but no, I preferred Daddy's arms. We all swam back together. One of my earliest memories is of those naive lifeguards trying to convince me their plastic float mobiles were safer than Dad.

He used to sing silly songs.

Put your shoes on Lucy
Don't you know you're in the city?
Put your shoes on Lucy
Don't you know it isn't pretty?
Lucy likes to be barefoot
wherever she goes
'cause she loves to hear the wiggle
of her toes.

And he was friendly. "Hello, how are you? What do you do? How long have you lived here?" to the waitress, the casual neighbor, the receptionist at the pool. Being young, I was easily embarrassed.

Still, everyone else's Dad was old and lumpy, big beer-belly and sloppy growth on his chin. I would die if I had to kiss a father like that good night! Me, I'd always have a Dad, and the best one too. A friend of mine used to make fun of my protective pride of my father. "My Daddy's the best damn enderkrednolojist in the whole wide world!" he used to whine in a bratty voice, and we'd laugh. In high school they "really got off on your Dad's accent, man." And when I brought a girlfriend home from college for vacation she couldn't stop telling me how good-looking he was. "I couldn't take my eyes off him. I hope he didn't notice," she said apologetically.

Some evenings are wonderful. Wayne and Eve Bower were over and we were talking about United States involvement in Chile, medical confidentiality and the law (Mom had just presented a seminar), and Wayne Williams' trial in Atlanta. We all agreed that he probably was guilty but they didn't have the goods. They were dragging witnesses in off the streets, trying to prove he was gay. "He's not on trial for homosexuality!" Mom said. Dad was quiet the whole time, then he summed it all up for us. "It's the kind of thing, when you can't score a goal, move the goal post."

Then, we were pulling Dad's shirt off, tugging at his arms, already loose and fragile in their sockets, and I said, "Gosh, what we do to you . . ." "Don't be silly," he said. "It's what you do for me." We got him on the bed and he rolled the wrong way and there he was crumpled on his face and he started laughing. "How can you laugh?" "It's a lot better, when you think of the alternative," he said.

As I reach the end of this book I realize I am anxious. I don't like the end of this story. I run my bath water, and in the slurping and swirling I hear "Roni! Roni!" It's my mother calling and I run out to the stairs. Quiet. My imagination. There's no emergency.

Tony Perlman's daughter Ellen told me that after Tony's last visit he was telling Patsy about it and she got very upset. "Don't get upset," he said, "because it wasn't depressing. It was uplifting. It was an uplifting experience to see that David, going through all he's going through, can still be himself, with the same spirit as always."

November 1983

I haven't written in a long time—a good sign, I suppose. I am at peace with myself; the whole family is more resolved. Up until a few months ago we were all knotted up in anger and hurt, like a gold chain left in the back of a drawer that has become so tangled up you don't even know where to begin to unravel it. But we're at peace now, even—to the extent possible—at peace with the raging illness. We are living with a beast, but we are ruining all the beast's fun because we do not give in to it. We think, we talk, we even laugh; most of all, we love. The beast has not taken our love, which would be its ultimate triumph.

January 1984

Physically, Dad's situation has deteriorated. He had an elective gastrostomy several months ago, when swallowing became difficult and dangerous. Then four months later we had to rush him to the hospital for an emergency tracheotomy. He just started choking and spitting and coughing one day, and we had to call an ambulance and make a split-second decision en route to the hospital. So we feed him by tube, and we've all learned how to suction out his bronchi and clean his air passages. We keep a close eye on him, and he seems to have adjusted fairly well. As long as he's on a plateau he's okay. He's so patient, he can adjust to anything. I used to think not being able to speak would be devastating to him. But we can still read his lips, and if he has something important to say he uses the computer. I think the times that were hardest on him were the days when he was continually losing functions: the arms, then the fingers, slowly the voice—requiring constant readjustment, mourning of the loss, then adjusting anew. But now he seems resolved. He knows what he has and what he's lost. He focuses on what he has: ears for music and radio news and stories we tell; eyes for loved ones, books and TV sports (a new interest he's developed); an active mind that still unravels research mysteries; skin for touching; an occasional gentle parting of the lips in a kiss; and eyebrows for activating the single switch on the computer. The original computer had been designed for a woman who, though aphasic, still controlled movement of her jaws. She activated the computer by biting on a mouth switch. But that was out of the question for David—his mouth was too weak. Bill Tracy, one of the guys who helped us figure out how the computer worked, took one look at David's eyebrows and realized their potential. He attached the switch to a sun visor that fits snugly around David's head. Now with a single arching of the brows, David can tell the cursor where to stop, which letter to select, which word to use, which phrase to bring out. Then he can either print it out on the printer or "speak" with his electronic voice synthesizer. He uses the computer for everything. It came ready with a vocabulary, but he has inserted his own words—"scrupulous," "propitious," "insulin," "secretions." There is also a list of phrases he can select from. "Hello how are you" for when people come to visit, "Please come again soon" for when they leave. And for people hearing the voice synthesizer for the first time there is, "How do you like my accent," said in the computers inimitable style. When Willis Williams leaves in the morning Dad flashes him a "You keep out of meanness." And he has a whole list of famous Humphrey Bogartisms. "Was you ever bitten by a dead bee?" And then, specialized phrases for family members. Like "Patience is a virtue, Michael"—a warning about Michael's temper. Or, "Leora, speak up I can't hear you" for Leora, not exactly known for whispering. And then the bare necessities: "I need a trach suction," "Hey, what about my lunch?" and so on.

Even when he's not using the computer, he lets his eyebrows do the talking. When a friend walks into the room, the eyebrows go up and down, up and down. "Hello, hello." Or if he agrees with what you're saying, the eyebrows start going. "Right on. I agree one hundred percent. Terrific." It's amazing how much energy he exudes through the furrows in his forehead and those bright blue eyes, even while the rest of his body sits small and motionless in that chair. Even now, when he is completely paralyzed and cannot even speak, swallow, or chew, he is a center of energy, serene and light.

Sometimes we think he could live forever like this. He shows no sign of failure. He has even started going in to work now. Once a week, he and Mr. Williams get on the special city transport van for the handicapped and drive into Vanderbilt. At the hospital Dad meets with his lab workers and listens in on the endocrine meetings. He doesn't say a word, but when he gets home he sits down at the computer and writes a long letter with his comments, suggestions, advice.

"He'll outlive all of us in the end," Mom says.

And Leora, never one to miss a good one-liner, chimes in. "He better not—he won't have anyone to take care of him if he does."

August 1984

A lot of changes are in store for our little family.

It's scary. We're all leaving home.

Dana completed her freshman year at Vanderbilt University last year, and now Leora—the baby of the family and the last one at home—is also starting college there. I am going up to New York City to do graduate work at the Columbia University School of Journalism. And Michael is settled into a high-geared, fast-paced consulting job in Greenwich, Connecticut.

Which leaves Mom alone to hold the fort, to care for Dad, to suction him and feed him and bathe him and love him.

Can we leave the two of them? I don't know, I ask myself that question all the time, thinking that at the last moment I'll unpack my bags, to hell with Columbia and stay here in Nashville. But I can see David flinch even at my mere entertainment of the option. He wants my life to go on; he wants all of us to learn and grow. He appreciates how much I have learned during my two years at the newspaper here—he is always pointing out what I've done, insisting on seeing every article, reading every word—but he knows I'm ready for a new challenge. After all, he's the appreciator of excellence, always bidding us to push ourselves, to do our best, attain the highest. I remember when I got the acceptance letter from Columbia and called home. Mr. Williams, the nurse, answered the phone. "Just tell my father I got in," I told him. A few minutes later Mr. Williams picked up the phone again, and said, "Your father says, 'terrific.'" And I could see it. I could visualize the little exchange, how David's eyes must have lit up as he raised his eyebrows and mouthed 'terrific.'

And then there's Dana. Proof incarnate of how important Normal Living really is. She lived on campus last year, Hemingway Dormitory, second floor. Just five minutes from home, but it was a different world, a world of frat parties and bull sessions and friends all over, down the hall and upstairs and across the quad. She really came out of herself. She shimmered. The college Dana was different from the high school Dana: livelier and much more extroverted, with a touch of silliness and giddiness. We couldn't keep track of all the boys' names she mentioned: Rick, Bob, Jim, Thomas. We couldn't reach her on the telephone—she was always out, never in her room. She made lots of friends, and one best friend in particular. She also made the Dean's list.

And throughout the school year she came home, visiting regularly, her schedule synchronized with that of Leora and Pauline to give them maximum flexibility. And every time she was home she slipped back into the routine easily; remembering Dad's afternoon snack at four, his favorite TV show—M*A*S*H—at five, and a little rundown on college life after the evening news.

Michael's career also shot off like a rocket. Sure, he could have gotten a job in Nashville. I'm sure a Harvard MBA can get a job pretty much wherever he or she wants. But Michael didn't want just any old job, and just any job wasn't what David wanted for Michael either. What Michael's doing now is really top-notch, high-caliber stuff. I don't pretend to understand it and besides, he's not at liberty to discuss his "cases." But he jets around the country, tie carefully selected to match his pressed shirt and jacket, making three or four cities in two or three days and working nights and early mornings and weekends. Moving from cozy little Cambridge to the competitive world of professional business was difficult, but he made it.

All in all, Leora was the star last year. I had struck out on my own and was living in a little apartment not far from home at Timber Lane, where Leora was staying with Mom and Dad. You'd think that much responsibility would grate on a seventeen-year-old kid, but not on Leora. She did everything with grace. "Grace under pressure," Ernest Hemingway's definition of courage. Leora was tough but always sensitive, practical but very gentle. Mom could count on her. Mom always knew that if Leora said she would be home at three, she'd be there on the dot. If Leora said she'd take care of dinner, she'd scrape something together and have the table set by the time Mom walked in the door. What's more, she did all that while making straight A's and being a dynamite class president. In May, Michael flew down and the six of us—including Dad, suction bottles and all—trooped off to Leora's high school graduation. Tzur Fabian, my Israeli cousin who is living in Florida, also joined us. It was beautiful, and our kid sister walked away with one of the most coveted prizes of all, the Civitan Award. Considering all the extra burdens Leora coped with, it was incredible. Need I say it? Dad was thrilled. He had sworn to live to see Leora graduate, and he'd made it.

I think Dad also gets a kick out of the fact that Leora's going to take the pre-medical track in college. Last summer she worked in Dad's lab conducting sperm counts. She seems to have a knack for chemical equations and double helixes. So it looks like we'll finally get a doctor out of this bunch . . .

Still, this fall will be a big adjustment. Dad is worried, I can tell. He smiles less readily and often appears to be deep in thought; in notes and messages he uses the word "burden." Mom is also tense. She is probably terrified but she would never say so; she would never try to discourage us from going on with our lives.

Instead, she tries to figure out ways to cope: she will get more nursing help for the late afternoons and weekends. But she does not want a live-in nurse—she is adamant on this point. I used to think it was just some bull-headed idea she'd gotten in her head. But now I understand why. This is her way of saying she does not want someone else to take over. That this is her responsibility, her commitment. That she is with David; she will always be with him, they are going it together. She is his companion, his live-in. She wants to be in that role—the two of them together, a couple bonded, man and wife until the end.

And they are. It's amazing. On Saturday mornings when the two of them sleep in late, Mom crawls out of her covers and up onto Dad's hospital bed and snuggles up close to him. I knock on the door and open it a crack to find two love birds tangled up with one another. Dad's bony arms and thighs are hidden under the blankets; all I see are his pale blue eyes shining as Mom kisses his forehead. An optical illusion: all is well. I want to take a picture, frame the two of them together.

I think we were all a little bit worried that Dad would feel he had accomplished all his objectives once Leora graduated. But don't worry: he has already set new goals. He's just applied for a new grant to continue the male contraceptive research, and he is proofreading the final draft of the book he and Mom co-edited, *To Provide Safe Passage*, a collection of essays on the humanistic side of medical care. The project grew out of the overwhelming response to our article in the *New England Journal of Medicine*. To my parents, the reaction signaled a need. It indicated not only a gap in medical training but also a dearth in the literature. So David and Pauline decided to expand on the ideas in that article with a collection of essays written by a variety of people—both lay and professional—about a spectrum of issues, from senile dementia to cancer. At times David has said that, all his scientific research notwithstanding, this may be his greatest contribution to the medical field. The project had the additional bonus of allowing my parents the opportunity to work together, combining their writing and medical skills in a joint effort. Working together has added a whole new dimension to their relationship: a new dialectic give-and-take, a new exploration and sharing, a new togetherness. It's interesting to watch the dynamics: Mom wants to goof off but David insists they get to work; then David gets tired and Mom stays up until late at night to figure something out.

Meanwhile, the search for a male Pill continues. It's not easy. After the first round of tests caused temporary impotence in some of the volunteers, Dad tried supplementing the LHRH analogue with the male hormone, testosterone. No side effects this time, but they were back to square one: the volunteers' sperm count didn't drop as drastically as it should have. So they increased the dose of analogue, infusing it through a small pump that works continuously. Those results "look quite good," says Dad, the ever-cautious scientist, on his computer. The goal now: to refine the system so the contraceptive can be given just once a month, in the form of an injection. One thing is clear: it's going to take a long time to get it right.

People often ask me what I've learned from Dad, what his message to the world is. And I often wonder how he does it. "He's amazing," I say. And friends respond, "That's an understatement."

If I had to write a formula, I'd say: start with a base of normal living. Reminds me of a story. Stan flew down to visit recently with his six-year-old son Oren. After just a little hesitancy, Oren got along famously with Dad, drawing him pictures and telling him all about dinosaurs. When he went back home a friend of Stan's said, "I heard you went to visit a very sick man this weekend." "No," Oren answered, "David isn't sick. He just can't move. But he isn't sick."

Add to that, one part creativity. Every morning when Dad gets up he gets himself hooked on to the computer. Sometimes for an hour or two, sometimes for eight or ten hours straight. This man has things to do, ideas to express, letters to write, stories to tell. He has direction and a sense of purpose. Seated at his computer he might as well be at a desk in an office anywhere in the world. He is not just a man in a wheelchair desperate to communicate— he is a person carrying on a life. With a little help from Radio Shack.

And with a little help from a loving family. Yes, add lots of love—one part, two parts, six parts love. Incoming and outgoing. There is little doubt in any of our minds that had Dad been forced to go into a nursing home he would never have survived this long. We're lucky: we've been able to handle the medical care. Mom's a doctor, the children are the right ages. But more than medical care, it's love. After washing up and suctioning, there is a kiss, a hand on the forehead, "Anything else you need, sir?" The love goes both ways: when Mom fell and hurt her wrist, Dad typed out a note on his computer: Roni—buy rose for Mom—card say I'm sorry and all my love.

Add a healthy sense of self-esteem. And under no circumstances allow even an ounce of self-pity. Regrets inevitably seep into the mixture, but try your damnedest to contain them. Dad still sees himself as a part of the world. Rather than focus on the hundreds of activities from which he is excluded, he keeps his eyes and ears open to the world. He can go to the hospital. He can visit with people. He knows more about what's going on around Nashville, from the radio, than any of us. And he gets involved, writing letters to the editor, commentaries on the twentieth century. He has something to say for himself; he doesn't hold back.

Don't forget a good sense of humor. We had a fright a few weeks ago. Dad thought he was losing his hearing. Kept asking us to turn the volume up on the television, said there was a ringing buzz in his ears. But then we discovered the cause: ever since his illness, he's had very oily skin and abnormal wax build-ups in his ears. One night we went in with Q-tips and lo and behold—pulled out reams of wax. Now he can hear! So remember, when you don't know whether to laugh or cry, laugh. The best thing is always to laugh.

Add a pinch of obstinacy, six pints of wisdom, and infinite patience. So that when he needs something and he mouths his request, and we don't understand, and he mouths it again and we still don't understand; he will mouth it again, or try another combination of words, or spell it out . . . until we understand. And then we discover that he is sitting on his hand, poor thing, but he's not mad about it.

Finally, add one magical part of special essence. Find it in beautiful young children, in wise old men, on the grass on a dew-laden summer morning. I have no idea where it comes from. Maybe it's alchemy, using the ingredients mentioned above. It's a certain strength, a certain transcendence. Sometimes I think he must have an extra chemical, superfluous endorphins. I ask him, "What's your secret?" He doesn't answer, just smiles and looks at me with those glittering blue eyes. "C'mon Dad, what's your secret?" He smiles and mouths, "There is no secret." I stomp my feet, "Hey, you promised. You promised you'd tell me." But he just smiles as if to say, "One day you'll realize you understand."

I remember what he always used to say: Life is too short to be unhappy. Life is too short to fight with the ones you love. Enjoy every day, every hour. If you are listening to a piece of music, hear every note and every sound. If you are working on a paper, make it the best paper. If you are loving, love to the fullest, give it all you've got and don't hold back. And if it's a question of choosing between laughing or crying—laugh. Always laugh.

Normal Living.

Epilogue

David died on October 26, 1984.

During the last few months of his life he had grown perceptibly weaker. He required almost constant trach suctioning, was increasingly uncomfortable, and had great difficulty sleeping. Still, he managed to be productive and kept a smile on his face. In the year and a half since his tracheotomy, he had enjoyed visits from Pauline's sister from Israel, and from other friends from Australia and Europe. Thanks to the Words Plus computer, he and Pauline completed their book, *To Provide Safe Passage,* a collection of essays on the humanistic aspects of medical care. David also authored several scientific articles, essays about the marvels of the computer, and a wide array of letters, commentraies, limericks and poems on subjects ranging from politics to etiquette. Every Wednesday, accompanied by Mr. Williams, David went to work at the hospital. The Wednesday before he died was the first Wednesday in over fourteen months that he had failed to appear at the university. He left behind a long letter to his research team, in which he outlined experiments and made suggestions to take them through at leave five years of future research.

When David was buried, Rabbi Zalman Posner, who had come to know him through his frequent visits, compared his life to the Torah, the Jewish Scripture. The Torah is a finite book with a beginning, middle, and end, and a limited number of chapters, verses, and words. Yet its significance and meaning, extended through continual study, interpretation, and meditation, can be made infinite. In the same way, Posner said, David's life was finite, but the lessons learned from it will reverberate forever.

213

Appendix

The symptoms of ALS differ markedly from patient to patient. I will describe the course of events in my illness. They will include all the symptoms of ALS, only the sequence may not coincide with your own.

A. *Stiffness and Weakness of the Lower Limbs*

My first symptoms were stiffness and slight weakness of the lower limbs. It is important to wear shoes that allow you to get about safely and comfortably. I found the Wallaby half-boot ideal; it is not heavy, yet splints the ankle and lessens the danger of falling. You will, nevertheless, feel unsteady and should be conscious of small steps and of uneven surfaces. Use your eyes and take advantage of rails. Be careful; nothing is worse than falling, as it always sets one back. Walking in bare feet is difficult; use a hard-sole slipper in the bedroom. A good walking stick can make a world of difference. It should be the correct length for you with a comfortable grip. A rubber attachment to the stick will help you keep your balance on slippery surfaces; hold the stick on the stronger side of your body. Have a trained person instruct you in its use. When foot-drop develops, plastic orthopedic appliances (orthotics) will make walking easier and safer. These are placed in the shoe and are adjusted to mold comfortably around your calves with Velcro straps. They provide permanent splinting of the weakened foot and greatly facilitate walking. Avoid sitting in low, soft chairs; choose high, straight-backed chairs with arms.

B. *Weakness of the Upper Limbs*

Weakness of the upper limbs may cause difficulty with many everyday tasks such as washing, eating, and writing. Use a light comb, spoon, toothbrush, and razor. A disposable razor is useful, and if fine hand movements are difficult, change to an electric toothbrush. A spoon with a ladle at right angles to the handle is easier to use than conventional cutlery. Dressing may be difficult; avoid hooks, buttons, and tight clothes. Dress in pull-over shirts and replace hooks with Velcro. Bathing presents considerable difficulty. If you have a shower stall, install rails for arm support and wear bath clogs to keep from slipping. The bath must always be considered treacherous; use a bath chair which functions hydraulically to avoid accidents (available from Whitaker's). We had our bath chair installed in a Jacuzzi, which is very relaxing and gives temporary relief from stiffness and cramps. There are two other important everyday events which pose problems: the toilet and the bed. An elevated toilet seat is helpful, particularly with a convenient handrail. An electric hospital bed makes getting in and out easier and will help you find your most comfortable position.

C. *Exercise During the Early Stages of ALS*

The value of exercise in ALS is unproven. Nevertheless, my personal view is that exercise is very useful both physically and, more importantly, emotionally. There is, however, one critical difference between the patient with ALS and a normal individual —the patient should stop before becoming fatigued. Swimming provides good all-round exercise and is relatively safe, but watch out for cramps. Another good way of exercising is with a stationary bicycle. To avoid becoming bored, watch TV or listen to the radio while you work out. Weights of two or four pounds will help build the upper limbs. A rubber ball for the hands strengthens the muscles of the fingers.

D. *When ALS Has Progressed*

When weakness is generalized, you may be able to remain mobile using crutches or a walker. However, you may fatigue yourself. I made this mistake by resisting the wheelchair far too long. The wheelchair is a means of maintaining independence; it can be powered electrically. There are vans available with a platform for getting the chair on and off easily. When muscle strength is low, it is best to accept help rather than struggle futilely with dressing, washing, eating, etc. This will only frustrate you and your family. Keep your strength for vital tasks including, very importantly, spending time with your family. When you sit in a wheelchair twelve or more hours a day, little things assume vital proportions. Sitting on a hard or uneven surface, having a paralyzed limb lying against steel, having one's underpants hitched up too high or one's head falling on one's chest, all can make one very miserable. Learn what is comfortable and insist on it. I use a firm cushion and eggbox padding. My arms rest on pillows, as does my head. The biggest danger is developing bed sores. This is said to be rare in ALS, but I can vouch for the fact that it occurs. The best therapy is prevention—sit on a doughnut ring; sleep on a ring with a sheepskin rug underneath. Rest your bottom by lying in bed on your side. Care of the skin is critical— always keep dry! Rub irritated areas with zinc oxide ointment. The skin breaks down when nutrition is poor. This may be the definitive sign that intake of food is dangerously low, and, as in my situation, a gastrostomy may become essential. Another very vulnerable area is the shoulder. When muscle wasting is severe, use slings and avoid letting your arms hang free. Fingers tend to cramp; get someone to straighten them periodically. Get a Hoya lift for moving from bed to chair and back. It is a fiendish-looking thing which I refused initially (and very stupidly), but it will spare your family's backs, and their nerves. When you lose the use of your hands, you will probably feel depressed. Ingenious ways have been found to overcome this handicap. The key is to avoid the natural impulse to become passive. All four limbs should be put through a full range of movement even when paralyzed; this prevents contractures and pain.

What about bowels? My personal experience has been chronic

constipation. I have required a laxative and an enema twice a week. Do not neglect your bowels. Nothing is as uncomfortable and unnecessary as impaction. Scrupulous attention will head off this problem.

E. *Automatic Page Turner and Other Ways of Staying Informed*

An automatic page-turner (from Bard Rehabilitation Aids) will allow you to read books independently. Get help with newspapers and magazines. While your voice is intact, dictate letters, etc. If you have difficulty, Mother Nature will help and you'll learn quickly. Necessity is the mother of invention. I will discuss the computer later. The Talking Library in many cities provides a radio with special programming for the handicapped. A tape recorder is available from the Library of Congress with a wonderful selection of tapes. Use the TV only as a last resort. It is so seductive and good for allaying anxiety, but it reinforces all your passive impulses.

F. *Problems with Eating*

I now come to the most frightening and distressing symptoms of ALS: difficulty with swallowing, speaking, and breathing. Problems with swallowing cause gagging, coughing, and a sensation of choking when food goes down the wrong way. The most important advice is to concentrate while you eat. Talk, laugh, and read, but not while you eat. I learned to avoid all citrus fruits and spicy foods. I drank orange juice with lots of sugar. I was able to tolerate soft-boiled eggs. In fact, for some months I was living proof of the incredible edible egg! I became fatigued when I had to chew large pieces of food on which I gagged. My family put food through the blender, and I handled this successfully for some months. As eating became more difficult, I began to skip meals. I got by on two eggs, orange juice, and a glass of milk to which was added ice cream and coffee. Even that was more than I could handle, and the resulting poor nutrition probably accounted for the bed sore. It was only after a particularly severe bout of choking and coughing that I belatedly agreed to have a gastrostomy. There are some who prefer an esophagostomy, an alterna-

tive to the gastrostomy in which a tube is inserted surgically into the esophagus. I, fortunately, had a wise, able, and practical surgeon who simply said, "You don't want to spend all day being fed. We can insert a large tube into your stomach and that means greater ease and rapidity of feeding and your tube won't clog!" I have been very grateful for his advice. The procedure was performed under local anesthesia, and there were moments of intense pain. After surgery, I was uncomfortable for a few days. Despite this, I recommend gastrostomy. Within a few days, I was on maintenance feeding. I use a preparation put out by Mead-Jonson called Isocal. I take seven cans a day (1750 calories). Initially, I was fed small amounts every hour, but now I am able to tolerate four daily feeds of about 600 ml (we add up to 250 ml of water to the Isocal.) What problems can you expect? There is a constant ooze around the gastrostomy site which must be dressed every day. The skin may become raw and tender from the ooze and from adhesive tape. We use alcohol to clean the ooze and rub well with cream and use only paper tape. The tube may fall out. This happened to me about a year after the operation but can be avoided by electively changing the tube every six months. The procedure is simple and the only mildly uncomfortable. It usually takes no more than five minutes because the body has prepared a tract around the old tube along which the new one readily passes. Infection is possible but rare. Some patients have diarrhea with certain food preparations. You may find the solution is simply to take a smaller volume more slowly; otherwise, try a different brand. Some patients describe a feeling of fullness along with weakness, nausea, and sweating. This is thought to be caused by rapid emptying of the stomach (the dumping syndrome). It is very unpleasant! I have only experienced this twice and both times when severely constipated. The only treatment is to switch to small frequent feeds given very slowly. Avoid constipation! Patients with ALS seem to be very sensitive to drugs that influence bowel action. I avoid them totally.

G. Problems with Breathing

As your muscles get weak, you may have trouble with breathing or more likely with coughing effectively to bring up the secretions from the lungs. This makes you susceptible to infection. Avoid contact with anyone with a cold, cough, or flu. We have found postural drainage helpful. This is performed by lying on your side with you head lower than your feet. Have someone tap on your chest. Secretions can become thick, cause severe distress, and be life-threatening. After such an experience, it is not difficult to opt for a tracheotomy. However terrifying this may sound, I had a tracheotomy in April 1983. The operation is short and painless, but there is discomfort with lots of gagging. The first two days after surgery are rough. You may require very frequent suction which can be uncomfortable. The quality of nursing is critical. I had outstanding care in Vanderbilt University's SICU (Surgical Intensive Care Unit). Your family will need education in handling what can best be called tracheotomy toilet. Make sure at least two people know the ropes and have all the supplies before you go home. We believe two suction machines should be on hand: one for mouth, the other for tracheotomy suction. Disposable catheters are best. We store them in sterile water and use them for no more than twenty-four hours. The dressing around the tube and the inner tube itself require daily changing and cleaning, respectively. The ribbon securing the tube must be kept clean and the opening covered with a moistened gauze. At first there is a tendency to use the suction excessively. Don't have suction every time there is a noise in your chest. You're the best judge of when you need suction. At night and in the morning use postural drainage. Have both machines available at all times because you will usually have many mouth secretions. You should have an oxygen tank at home. Use it whenever you feel breathless, especially after a rough bout of suction. We use the clean technique, washing the hands well before each suction. What was once terrifying becomes routine. Some problems may be encountered: infection is a threat; you may feel ill and secretions may develop a yellow color or become bloodstained. Call your doctor, who will prescribe medication. The tube can fall out; it can be replaced using an obturator. This is simply a rod which allows the tube to be inserted without injuring the trachea; it should always be available. I believe it is essential to purchase a generator. Otherwise, it is terrifying when the electricity fails. With a tracheotomy in place and difficulty in swallowing, mouth secretions tend to become more and more troublesome. When saliva pools in the mouth, it easily runs into the trachea causing gagging. I have had irradiation to my salivary glands, which has had a modest effect in reducing the amount of saliva I secrete.

H. *Problems with Communication*

After a tracheotomy, you lose mobility, but the most serious loss is speech. If your voice is strong the tube can be closed temporarily, which will enable you to speak. In my own case, my voice was so weak that the tracheotomy ended any useful speech. This means mouthing the words and relying on lip reading—slow and frustrating but possible! We then found out by serendipity that a computer was available which operates with a single switch. This makes it possible for ALS patients with only one working muscle to have a whole wonderful world reopen, a world that had seemed irretrievably lost. The computer is available from Words + Living Center. I communicate by typing messages on a screen. I use a special switch which attaches to my eyebrow muscle. Alternative switches can be developed to utilize any muscle group that has function. A printer prints on command (this paper was prepared entirely with the computer). A voice synthesizer enunciates the words and provides an alarm system when I need help. An electronic miracle!

I have described the tools which have enabled me to contend with the physical disabilities of ALS. However, these count for nought without the love, encouragement, emotional support, and devotion of my wife Pauline, my children, my family, and close friends. They have made possible the full expression of our credo for creeping paralysis—*cogito ergo sum*—I can think, therefore I'm able to function. When there is love, all life is worth the fight. In Dylan Thomas' words:

> Do not go gentle into that good night,
> Rage, rage against the dying of the light.

> —*David Rabin and Leora Rabin*

References

The following is a list of publications and associations we found particularly helpful:

Books

Cousins, Norman, *Anatomy of an Illness* (New York: W.W. Norton and Co.), 1979. Available in paperback from Bantam Books.

Graham, Jory, *In the Company of Others* (New York: Harcourt Brace Jovanovich), 1981.

Kübler-Ross, Elisabeth, *On Death and Dying* (New York: Macmillan Publishing Co.), 1969.

Lear, Martha Weinman, *Heartsounds* (New York: Pocket Books), 1980.

Rabin, David and Pauline, *To Provide Safe Passage* (New York: The Philosophical Library), 1985.

Simonton, Carl, *Getting Well Again* (New York: Bantam Books), 1980.

Associations

Muscular Dystrophy Association (the MDA covers many diseases, including ALS), 810 Seventh Ave., New York, New York 10019 (212) 586-0808

Amyotrophic Lateral Sclerosis Society of America (ALSSOA)
15300 Ventura Boulevard, Suite 315
PO Box 5951
Sherman Oaks, California 91403
(818) 990-2151

National Amyotrophic Lateral Sclerosis Foundation, Inc.
185 Madison Ave.
New York, New York 10016
(212) 679-4016

Words Plus (computers for the handicapped)
622 S. Fair Oaks Avenue
Sunnyvale, California 94086
(408) 730-9588